HEMORRHOIDS

HEMORRHOIDS

Sidney E. Wanderman, M.D.,
with Betty Rothbart, M.S.W.,
and the Editors of
Consumer Reports Books

CONSUMER REPORTS BOOKS
A Division of Consumers Union
Yonkers, New York

The ideas, procedures, and suggestions contained in this book are not intended to replace the services of a physician. All matters regarding your heath require medical supervision. You should consult with your physician before adopting any of the procedures in this book. Any applications of the treatments set forth in this book are at the reader's discretion, and neither the author nor the publisher assumes any responsibility or liability therefor.

Copyright © 1991 by Sidney E. Wanderman, M.D.

All rights reserved, including the right of reproduction in whole or in part in any form.

Library of Congress Cataloging-in-Publication Data
Wanderman, Sidney.
Hemorrhoids / by Sidney E. Wanderman with Betty Rothbart and the Editors of Consumer Reports Books.
p.   cm.
Includes index.
ISBN 0-89043-447-6
1. Hemorrhoids—Popular works. 2. Consumer education.
I. Rothbart, Betty. II. Consumer Reports Books. III. Title.
RC865.W3   1991
616.3'5—dc20   91-19547
CIP

Some of this material has been previously published in
THE HEMORRHOID BOOK
(1981), Grosset & Dunlap.

Design by GDS / Jeffrey L. Ward
First printing, November 1991
Manufactured in the United States of America

Hemorrhoids is a Consumer Reports Book published by Consumers Union, the nonprofit organization that publishes *Consumer Reports*, the monthly magazine of test reports, product Ratings, and buying guidance. Established in 1936, Consumers Union is chartered under the Not-For-Profit Corporation Law of the State of New York.

The purpose of Consumers Union, as stated in its charter, are to provide consumers with information and counsel on consumer goods and services, to give information on all matters relating to the expenditure of the family income, and to initiate and to cooperate with individual and group efforts seeking to create and maintain decent living standards.

Consumers Union derives its income solely from the sale of *Consumer Reports* and other publications. In addition, expenses of occasional public service efforts may be met, in part, by nonrestrictive, noncommercial contributions, grants, and fees. Consumers Union accepts no advertising or product samples and is not beholden in any way to any commercial interest. Its Ratings and reports are solely for the use of the readers of its publications. Neither the Ratings nor the reports nor any Consumers Union publications, including this book, may be used in advertising or for any commercial purpose. Consumers Union will take all steps open to it to prevent such uses of its materials, its name, or the name of *Consumer Reports*.

Dedicated
to my wife Jeannette,
my daughters Marcia and Lisa,
my son-in-law Bill,
and
my grandchildren Robin and Anthony

This book is for people who have suffered from hemorrhoids or other bowel problems—and for those who want to make sure they never will

Contents

■

Introduction		1
1	What Are Hemorrhoids?	5
2	A Short Course in Anatomy	9
3	What Causes Hemorrhoids?	15
4	Symptoms: Are You Sure Your Problem Is Really Hemorrhoids?	19
5	The Rectal Examination	29
6	Constipation: The Major Cause of Hemorrhoids	31
7	Diarrhea: The Traveler's Route to Hemorrhoids	43
8	For the Pregnant Woman	49
9	Special Problems of the Elderly	51
10	Self-Care of Hemorrhoids	55
11	How a Doctor Treats Hemorrhoids	63
12	How to Prevent Hemorrhoids	69
13	Flatulence	77

14	Itching: A Delicate Subject	83
15	Colitis and Diverticulitis	89
16	How a Doctor Treats Fissures, Fistulas, Polyps, and Colon-Rectal Cancer	95
17	Sexually Transmitted Diseases	101
18	Toilet Training: Helping Children Develop Healthy Bowel Habits	115
19	Anorectal Disorders in Children	123
Index		131

Introduction

Hemorrhoids and many other bowel problems can easily be prevented and treated. Yet because many people are embarrassed about discussing their bowels, they hesitate to seek medical treatment for rectal and intestinal problems. "Oh, I could never talk about that with my doctor," they say. Feeling ashamed or simply unable to articulate their complaints, they endure discomfort that could be relieved, and postpone consulting a doctor until pain or bleeding forces them to do so. As with any medical problem, it is best to seek medical care promptly because early treatment is usually simpler and more effective. And the sooner you see a doctor, the sooner your worst fears are often put to rest.

Let's declare a moratorium on embarrassment. Free yourself to learn how to keep bowels healthy, when to seek medical care, how to describe symptoms to your doctor, and how and when to use self-care methods.

One of the most prevalent rectal/bowel disorders in our society is hemorrhoids, the condition in which normal hemorrhoidal veins become enlarged, fill with blood clots, bleed, or protrude and cause discomfort. As many as half the people in the United States and other industrialized nations may suffer from them. The reason: fast-paced lifestyles and inadequate dietary regimes that promote poor bowel habits and result in hemorrhoids.

If you answer yes to any of the following questions, you are at risk for getting hemorrhoids.

- Are you an "eat and run" person at breakfast?
- Are you frequently constipated?
- Is "regularity" a problem for you?
- Does your diet consist mostly of meat and refined foods?
- Does your diet lack roughage such as bran and raw vegetables?
- Do you often postpone bowel movements until a more convenient time?
- Do you often take laxatives?

If you have hemorrhoids, there are many effective, easy, and inexpensive self-care methods you can use that are superior to various ointments you have seen advertised. But it is important to remember that although hemorrhoids are the best-known anal disorder, they are by no means the only one. Defer self-care until your doctor confirms that your problem is, in fact, hemorrhoids. Serious problems, even cancer, may have the same symptoms as hemorrhoids.

Nowhere is colon-rectal cancer more prevalent than in

the Western world. Every year the number of cases rises. According to the American Cancer Society, in the United States in 1977, 104,000 people were diagnosed as having colon-rectal cancer. In 1990, that figure rose to 155,000. Of these, 53,000 with colon cancer and 7,600 with rectal cancer will die. Those who are diagnosed earliest have the best chances of survival, with a five-year survival rate of 57 percent for those with colon cancer and 79 percent for those with rectal cancer.

Although not all causes of colon-rectal cancer are known, the Western diet may be one culprit. Westerners eat too many highly refined, low-residue foods processed with chemical additives, and too much animal protein and fat. People who eat less of these foods and more roughage may be less likely to develop colon-rectal cancer.

In addition to hemorrhoids and cancer, this book covers many other bowel problems, from infection, sexually transmitted diseases, and constipation and diarrhea to special problems of children, the elderly, and pregnant women. By becoming aware of all the possibilities, you can become alert to symptoms, less likely to dismiss them as "only hemorrhoids," and more attuned to the importance of early diagnosis and treatment, even if they are "only hemorrhoids."

Hemorrhoids and bowl disorders occur among people in every walk of life. As former chief proctologist at a corporate health diagnostic center, I examined 10,000 people a year, from stenographers to corporation presidents. I would like to see all people assume an executive "take-charge" attitude toward the business of keeping their bodies healthy.

1

What Are Hemorrhoids?

■

Everyone has hemorrhoidal veins in the anal area called the hemorrhoidal plexus. When these normal veins become abnormally distended, they cause symptoms such as pain and bleeding. One theory is that an anatomical disadvantage predisposes the human species to hemorrhoids. Hemorrhoidal veins lack valves, which would help support the weighty column of blood that passes through them. But earlier in our evolution, when we walked on four legs like other mammals, we had no need for such support. Because the long axis of our body was parallel to the ground, the pull of gravity was more evenly distributed. When we learned to walk on two feet, the relationship of our body to gravity changed. The weight of the blood column now rested heavily in the veins of the lower rectum and anus, a burden these areas were ill-equipped to handle.

This theory explains that any *extra* pressure on these already overworked veins distorts their delicate structure

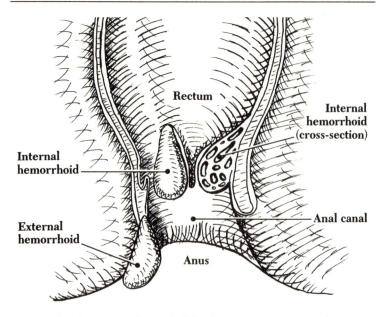

Hemorrhoids occur at the end of the digestive tract. Internal hemorrhoids originate in the rectum, external hemorrhoids near the anal opening. Covered by sensitive skin, external hemorrhoids are generally more painful.

and distends them into hemorrhoids. Some hemorrhoids are external. They can be felt with a finger and resemble soft swellings around the anal opening. Internal hemorrhoids, however, cannot be felt or seen, because they are hidden inside the anal canal.

If hemorrhoids are small, you may not even know you have any. They become troublesome when they increase in size, stretching the membrane of the vein wall. The membrane becomes thin. When feces pass from the body, they rub against hemorrhoids and irritate the increasingly flimsy membrane until it breaks and bleeds. Bleeding internal hemorrhoids may not be painful, because internal membranes lack pain-sensitive nerve fibers. External hemorrhoids, however, are covered by skin that is dense with pain nerves. Ulcerated or thrombosed external hemorrhoids can be excruciatingly painful.

Thrombosis is the lodging of a blood clot in a hemorrhoid. In an external hemorrhoid, the clot feels like a hard protrusion. If the clot is large, this condition can become especially painful. The clot may expand within the vein, stretching skin nerves and causing increasing pain. Doctors sometimes excise clots surgically, but clots often break out of the hemorrhoid spontaneously, slipping out of a break in the skin like a pea from a pod. Sometimes clots simply dissolve and pass out of the hemorrhoid to rejoin the blood flow.

Difficult passage of hard, dry stool may rub against an internal hemorrhoid and prolapse it—push it outside the anal opening. This sudden irritation may cause the anal sphincter muscles to go into spasm, trapping the hemorrhoid outside the anal canal. This painful condition usually can be eased with hot baths, and you can gently push the prolapsed internal hemorrhoid back inside the anal canal with a lubricated finger.

Many people misdiagnose anal bleeding. They may assume that it is caused by a hemorrhoid but find out later that the bleeding is a symptom of cancer. Or they may panic and assume they have cancer when the blood is really from a hidden internal hemorrhoid. *Any* bleeding from the anus, regardless of amount, should be checked by a doctor.

2

A Short Course in Anatomy

■

How would you draw the anatomy of the colon and rectum? Most people would draw a curving tunnel, with the anus as the exit. Yet they would omit some of the structures that make this area such an efficient, well-designed system for the elimination of body waste. The valves of Houston, for example, do not refer to Texas oil wells but are important parts of the rectum that perform a crucial anatomical function. Beneath the dentate line lie concealed clues to our ancient past. The anal sphincter muscles are powerful, for they stay in a steady state of contraction until they relax and stretch during defecation.

The digestive system really begins at the mouth and ends at the anus. Since this book is concerned with the elimination process, let's begin this anatomy lesson where a doctor begins an examination: at the anus and working upward (see Chapter 5).

The skin around the anal opening is slightly darker than

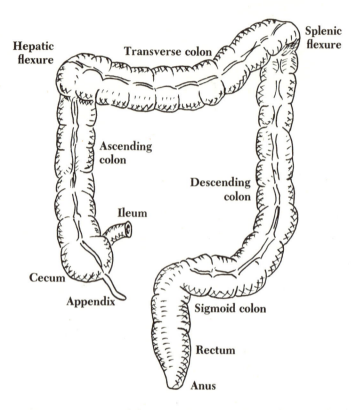

Diagram of the colon (the large intestine)

the rest of the skin. It contains sweat and sebaceous (grease) glands and hair follicles. Many nerve fibers make the anus both erogenous and extremely sensitive to pain.

The anal opening is an oval aperture an inch or so in front of the spine, closer to the front in a woman than in a man. It is about an inch in circumference, but the encircling sphincter muscles can stretch it to five or six times that size, then close it again so tightly that it appears corrugated and puckered, like the top of a drawstring purse. The anus and

A Short Course in Anatomy

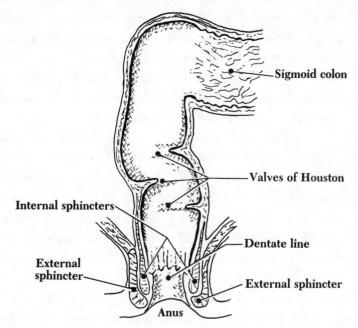

Diagram of the anus and rectum showing the internal and external sphincters and the valves involved in defecation.

the mouth—the two ends of the long digestive tract—are the only parts of the body capable of this pursing action.

Within the anal opening is the anal canal, less than two inches deep. The outermost quarter-inch is lined with skin. Muscles in the anal canal control the passage of feces out of the body.

At the top of the anal canal, the dentate line ridges the tunnel's walls. The dentate line is a ring of tissue folds, called papillae, arranged in a sawtooth design. Underneath the dentate line, between the papillae, lie hundreds of small glands, all vestigial. Earlier in our evolution, when we walked on all fours and sniffed at each other like dogs, the glands secreted aromatic sex juices that attracted mates.

Today the flasklike glands are empty. Like their better-known vestigial counterpart, the appendix, the glands are harmless unless they become infected or inflamed.

The dentate line marks the point where skin ends and membrane begins. About an inch beyond that, the tunnel widens and is now called the rectum. It is five or six inches long, extending upward with subtle bends and turns. The empty space within the rectum is called the lumen. Into it jut three fingerlike projections called the valves of Houston. The rectum is the last holding bin for feces on their way down through the tunnel. The valves of Houston serve as little shelves upon which feces rest between bowel movements. When the feces become heavy, the valves act like a trip mechanism, pressing against the rectal wall to send the signal that feces are ready to exit the body. This signal, which people experience as the urge to defecate, is also colloquially called the "call of nature." Medically, it is known as the final stage of the gastrocolic reflex. For children, learning to recognize the call of nature is key to toilet training. For adults, learning to respond to the call of nature and not postpone bowel movements is key to keeping the signal mechanism functioning smoothly.

At the top of the rectum the colon, or large intestine, begins. This six-foot-long organ, also known as the bowel, has four parts. The sigmoid colon, at the lowest end, is shaped like the letter S and begins at the upper part of the rectum. The sigmoid colon leads into the descending colon, a straight tube extending upward along the left side of the abdomen to the level of the lower left ribs. At this junction (the splenic flexure, or turn near the spleen) it meets the horizontal section of the colon called the transverse colon, which crosses the abdomen from left to right at about the level of an imaginary line three to four inches above the navel. Near the lower right ribs, at the liver, the transverse colon joins the ascending colon at the hepatic flexure (the turn near the liver). Like the descending colon, it is a vertical tube. The ascending colon actually starts at the cecum where the small intestines end and the appendix is attached. There is no digestion in the large intestine as in the small intestine. The fecal current is liquid at the cecum, and solid in the sigmoid colon. The large intestine removes water from the fecal current.

3

What Causes Hemorrhoids?

■

Many types of pressure can cause hemorrhoids:

- *Forcing a bowel movement.* Hemorrhoids are most commonly caused by pushing too hard and too long during a bowel movement, often because of constipation, diarrhea, or unhealthy bowel habits.
- *Heredity.* If many people in your family have troublesome hemorrhoids, it may be due to an inherited structural weakness of the vein walls that makes them unable to tolerate strains that other people can handle easily. Such strains can include jobs that require standing for long periods of time.
- *Holding breath during physical exertion.* Manual laborers and weight lifters who habitually strain often suffer hemorrhoids as a result of the Valsalva maneuver, a physiological reflex named after an eighteenth-century Italian doctor. If you grunt while lifting a heavy

object, you are holding your breath. This closes the glottis, forces all air downward, and causes the diaphragm to descend, pushing down other organs like a stick in a churn or a piston in an engine, and exerting sudden pressure on hemorrhoidal veins. During physical labor or exercise workouts, keep breath flowing. Concentrate on coordinating rhythmic inhaling and exhaling with your movements. Yoga is especially good for learning to do this.
• *Pregnancy.* Pregnancy can exert pressure on hemorrhoidal veins.
• *Psychological factors that increase straining during bowel movements.* Many people—overweight or not—suffer from hemorrhoids because subconsciously they try to punish themselves anally for overindulging orally. After overeating, they may feel so guilty or disgusted that they try to excrete the food quickly in the mistaken belief that doing so will prevent the calories from turning into fat. Of course, the digestive process cannot be speeded up this way. Such straining and pushing can cause hemorrhoids.

Many people subconsciously regard defecation as a symbolic as well as a physical act, associating it with issues of power, letting go, vulnerability, even mortality. In *The Denial of Death,* Ernest Becker wrote of a tribe that regards defecation as an act so undignified that they choose to deny its existence:

> Men of the Chagga tribe wear an anal plug all their lives, pretending to have sealed up the anus and

not need to defecate. . . . To say that someone is "anal" means that someone is trying extra-hard to protect himself against the accidents of life and danger of death, trying to use the symbols of culture as a sure means of triumph over natural mystery, trying to pass himself off as anything but an animal.

Too few people regard defecation as simply the end product of a wondrously efficient digestive system that retains nutrients and discards waste. A 93-year-old man whose ability to defecate was restored after successful surgery for colon cancer was unabashed in his feeling of relief. "It's like heaven," he said. "My bowels work again."

Psychotherapy can help uncover emotional causes for constipation and related problems. But on your own you can develop sensitivity to your body and keep from straining. Concentrating on breathing while sitting on the toilet can focus attention inward and promote the relaxation that is essential to healthy, normal bowel movements. Developing body awareness can prevent useless straining and also allow you the freedom to leave the toilet without defecating if you obey your body's signals that the time is not right.

Fostering awareness is not always easy. Society often conditions us to regard defecation as a dirty or negative part of life—something that merits disgust, not calm attention. But the rewards of such awareness can be relief of constipation and hemorrhoids, and an overall sense of lessened tension.

4

Symptoms: Are You Sure Your Problem Is Really Hemorrhoids?

■

For nearly two weeks, John, a tailor, experienced a stabbing pain whenever he passed gas or moved his bowels. He assumed he had hemorrhoids and applied an ointment every few hours. But it did not help. Finally the pain became so severe that John went to a proctologist, who found a sewing needle embedded in the lining of the anal canal. He removed it under local anesthetic—and John stopped holding needles and pins in his mouth when he sewed. (The same problem has occurred with toothpicks, chicken and fish bones, and even diaper pins.)

It is amazing that the needle traveled through the entire digestive tract before causing trouble; it is not at all amazing that John assumed that hemorrhoids caused his pain. Many people assume that just about any anal or rectal malady indicates hemorrhoids, simply because hemorrhoids are so common. Preparations claiming to relieve hemorrhoids are among the most widely advertised over-the-counter products.

But such assumptions can be dangerous. Pain, bleeding, and other symptoms may indicate other disorders and should be diagnosed by a physician. The more specific you can be in describing symptoms, the easier your doctor will find it to make an accurate diagnosis. For example, there are different types of pain and varying degrees of bleeding.

COMMON SYMPTOMS OF PROBLEMS IN THE LOWER BOWEL OR RECTUM

Pain is the most frequent reason people consult a proctologist. Most commonly, pain is felt right at the anal opening or just inside the anal canal, because these areas contain pain-sensitive nerve fibers. Because the rectum lacks these pain nerves, it cannot give such clear signals for help. It may, however, cause "referred" pain in the lower back, sex organs, bladder, or sciatic nerve. Referred pain highlights the need for a proctological examination along with every routine physical checkup.

Hemorrhoids are generally not painful. Hemorrhoidal pain arises from irritation, thrombosis, or spasm that traps a prolapsed internal hemorrhoid outside the anal opening. The anal sphincter muscles can go into spasm because of irritation from a crack in the membrane lining the canal, an abscess, an inflammation, or a foreign body.

A sharp, cutting pain that comes on with defecation, or sudden, darting pains that occur in the intervals between stool passage, may be caused by an anal fissure, a crack

Symptoms: Are You Sure Your Problem Is Really Hemorrhoids?   21

or tear in the skin around the anal opening or in the anal canal.

Tenderness and aching, particularly around the anal opening, are usually caused by early abscess formation or a fistula, a type of infection. Tenderness in the anal canal can indicate inflammation or ulceration, such as from syphilis or a scratch from a foreign object.

When describing pain to your doctor, indicate

- the type of pain
- the time of its onset in relation to bowel movements
- when you first noticed the pain

Until you see your doctor, relieve pain with hot sitz baths, acetaminophen, and stool softeners.

Bleeding may indicate a hemorrhoid, cancer, ulcer, or injury (such as a fissure). Always report bleeding to a doctor. Profuse bleeding may cause anemia. The type of bleeding sometimes indicates the most likely origin. *Bright red blood* comes from inside the anal canal. It may indicate hemorrhoids but not always. *Dark blood* has traveled farther within the colon and has lost oxygen along the way. The color of the blood is, therefore, important to report, but only a doctor can determine at what level the bleeding originated.

When describing bleeding to your doctor, indicate

- the blood's color (bright red or dark)
- the amount of bleeding
- whether bleeding occurs before, during, and/or after defecation

- whether you find blood on toilet paper, in the toilet bowl, mixed in with stool, or leaking onto underclothing
- whether discharge of pus or mucus occurs along with bleeding

All these symptoms, except for discharge of pus or mucus, may indicate hemorrhoids.

Until you see your doctor, relieve bleeding with ice and by pressing gauze or cotton padding on the anal opening.

Discharge of mucus or pus is caused by irritation of the bowel at any level. Pus or a mucous, watery, or bloody discharge usually comes from an abscess that has broken, a fistula, parasites, a tumor, inflammatory bowel disease, cancer, or sexually transmitted disease. Sometimes, however, a discharge is actually just moisture from heat or friction.

When describing a discharge to your doctor, indicate

- whether the discharge is bloody, watery, or contains mucus or pus
- whether you have diarrhea that is sometimes bloody and contains mucus
- whether the discharge comes from a slight protuberance around the anal opening or anal canal
- whether the discharge is accompanied by tenderness or aching

Until you see your doctor, catch any profuse discharge with gauze or cotton padding.

A *change in bowel habits*—persistent constipation, persistent diarrhea, or the two alternating—can indicate tension, poor diet, emotional stress, a tumor, or other disease. It is not unusual for constipation and diarrhea to occur during such traumatic experiences as divorce, the death of a loved one, or the loss of a job. As emotions calm, the body begins to function normally again.

When describing change in bowel habits to your doctor, indicate

- whether bowel movements are notably more or less frequent than usual
- whether you suffer persistent constipation, diarrhea, or the two alternating
- whether bowel movements result in the passage of gas only, not stool

A change from normal stool refers to a consistent narrowing of the stool, a change of stool color, or blood with the stool. Any of these may indicate the presence of a tumor; pale stool often occurs with diseases involving the bile ducts, including gallstones, or, less often, hepatitis.

In order to be aware of a change of stool, you need to know what "normal" stool means for you. This varies among individuals and is determined by diet, digestive process, strength of peristaltic contractions (undulation of the bowel wall necessary for defecation), and width of the rectum.

A healthy person's stool is formed, and yellow to brown in color. A black, tarry stool may indicate intestinal bleeding or cancer, but it may also be black from excess iron intake, spinach, or licorice. Beets can make the stool reddish.

When describing a change from normal stool to your doctor, indicate

- whether the stool has narrowed into a pencillike shape
- the presence of black, tarry stool or passage of blood, pus, or mucus with stool
- when you first noticed the change
- whether you experience cramping or fatigue

Swelling usually indicates a hemorrhoid, but it may also be a sign of infection.

When describing swelling to your doctor, indicate

- whether the swelling is accompanied by pain, bleeding, or discharge
- whether the swelling is constant or increases each day
- whether the swelling goes away, only to return with the next bowel movement

Until you see your doctor, relieve swelling with hot sitz baths.

Itching may be caused by hemorrhoids, allergy, parasites, antibiotics, emotional stress, skin disease, or diabetes.

When describing itching to your doctor, indicate

- whether the itching is worse at night
- whether itching occurs or worsens after eating certain foods
- whether you have been taking antibiotics
- whether you are under emotional stress
- when the itching started

Until you see your doctor, relieve itching with hot sitz baths and by applying petroleum jelly, calamine lotion, or witch hazel.

Protrusions from the anal canal are usually external hemorrhoids or prolapsed internal hemorrhoids that are pushed out of the anal canal and can sometimes be pushed back in.

A hard, rounded protuberance that occurs suddenly may be caused by a blood clot in an external hemorrhoid. Other types of protrusions may be low-lying polyps (growths), cancer, or the prolapsed wall of the anorectal canal (procidentia), which looks like a sleeve turned inside out.

When describing protrusions to your doctor, indicate

- the presence of bleeding or discharge
- when you first noticed it

Elevations around the anal opening, where skin may lack its normal, smooth feeling, may be caused by abscesses, fistulas, warts, herpes blisters, syphilis chancre, or even grease glands that have become plugged up to form whiteheads.

When describing elevations to your doctor, indicate

- whether the elevation increases in size each day
- whether there is pain or tenderness
- the presence of bleeding or discharge

Soilage is usually the result of weakened sphincter muscles or a tumor.

Symptom	When to see your doctor
Pain	Persistent pain Sharp, tearing pain with bowel movement
	Throbbing pain or tenderness
	Spasm
Bleeding	Any bleeding, regardless of amount
Discharge	Yellow, white, watery, or bloody discharge from anal opening or surrounding skin
Change in bowel habits	Persistent constipation, diarrhea, or the two alternating
	Desire to move bowels with passage only of gas or discharge
Change from normal stool	Consistent narrowing of stool to pencillike shape
	Black, tarry stool or blood passed with stool
Swelling	If accompanied by pain, bleeding, discharge, or progressively intense throbbing
Itching	If persistent and not relieved by self-care methods
Protrusions or elevations	Always see a doctor for diagnosis
Soilage	Uncontrollable leakage of feces

May indicate	Comments
Thrombosed hemorrhoid, fissure	Relieve pain with hot sitz baths, stool softeners, acetaminophen.
Abscess, fistula	Relieve pain with hot sitz baths until you see a doctor.
Trapped hemorrhoid, foreign object	Relieve pain with hot sitz baths.
Hemorrhoid, cancer, ulcer, injury	May cause anemia if profuse. Relieve with ice and padding until you see a doctor. Self-treat for hemorrhoids only after a doctor's diagnosis.
Abscess, fistula, venereal disease, cancer, parasites	Self-care not advised. Inform sexual partner if you suspect venereal disease.
Emotional stress, poor diet, cancer, other disease	Diminished emotional stress should ease symptoms.
Cancer, colitis, proctitis	Condition possibly not significant if happens rarely; see a doctor if it becomes habitual.
Cancer, inflammatory bowel disease	Know what "normal" stool is for you so that you can detect changes.
Cancer, hemorrhoid, disease of upper intestine or stomach—e.g. ulcers, diverticulosis, other gastrointestinal bleeding	Black stool may be caused by iron supplements, spinach, or licorice. Beets may cause reddish stool.
Hemorrhoid, abscess, fistula	Usually means hemorrhoid. Relieve with hot sitz baths until you see a doctor.
Allergy, parasites, emotional stress, skin disease, diabetes, or unknown origin	Self-care not advised *if* itching is chronic or severe. Relieve with hot sitz baths, petroleum jelly, calamine lotion, or witch hazel until you see a doctor.
Hemorrhoid, prolapse, cancer, abscess, fistula, warts, herpes, whiteheads	
Weakened sphincter muscles, tumor, impacted stool	Strengthen muscles with "buttock press" exercise (see page 75); see a doctor if condition does not improve in one month.

ALWAYS TELL YOUR DOCTOR:

- When you first noticed a symptom
- Whether you have ever experienced it before
- If there is bleeding or discharge
- If you have noticed any change in bowel habits or normal stool
- Whether a symptom appeared or worsens with a bowel movement
- The severity of your discomfort (Did you need to stay home from work?)
- Any self-treatment you used, and its result
- Whether you have had anal intercourse

WATCH OUT FOR THE WARNING SIGNALS OF COLON-RECTAL CANCER:

- Bleeding, any amount
- Blood passed with stool, or, less often, black, tarry stool
- Change in bowel habits
- Narrow, pencillike stool
- Abdominal cramping
- Persistent urge to defecate with passage only of gas or discharge
- Unaccustomed feeling of weakness
- Soilage associated with spasm
- Firm protrusion from the anal opening
- Persistent ulcer in skin alongside the anal opening

5

The Rectal Examination

■

"This is a very unflattering position," protests one patient.

"Why the hell would you want to do this for a living?" mutters another.

And before the examination even begins, another pleads, "Why don't we just call it a day?"

Many people dread the proctological examination. They postpone it countless times, cancel it at the last minute, or try to avoid even thinking about it. They say it is embarrassing, painful, disgusting, and a waste of time unless you are in pain or bleeding.

Sometimes their doctors join them in delaying the examination. Medical schools provide excellent training to their students but do not stress learning the technique of a complete proctological examination. In fact, some doctors never use the most basic proctological instruments and may never make use of their knowledge of rectal anatomy. These physicians share their patients' aversion to the rectal examination. So they advocate an annual physical checkup but neglect to include examination of the rectum as part of the procedure.

The fact remains, however, that of the thousands of cases of colon-rectal cancer reported each year, those that are detected early have a better chance for complete removal and cure. The examination is a small price to pay for the great benefit of early diagnosis or the relief of knowing you do not have cancer. To be safe, you should be sure a rectal examination is part of every general physical examination.

For most people the examination does not reveal serious disease. It is not a painful process, although there may be some discomfort. Relaxing helps. So does a "don't fight it, but join it" attitude. Most important, remember that the doctor examines you to help you, not to punish you.

By learning what the examination involves, you should even be able to use it as an opportunity to gain understanding of your body and how it works.

A NOTE FOR WOMEN

Women should try to schedule the examination between menstrual periods. If this is not possible, and if you are wearing a tampon, tell the doctor. Also inform the doctor if you have an intrauterine device (IUD). Tampons, IUDs, even forgotten diaphragms can be felt through the rectal wall. There have been instances when they were misread as growths.

BEFORE THE EXAMINATION BEGINS

Cleansing the bowel in preparation for sigmoidoscopy or colonoscopy makes it easier for the doctor to see inside you, and it is more comfortable for you. The examining doctor may recommend such measures as an enema, a liquid diet prior to the exam, or a laxative.

The proper position for a rectal examination varies from physician to physician. Many doctors have a patient lie on the left side. Or your doctor may ask you to kneel on a table with your shoulder and the side of your face on the table. This positions the rectum and sigmoid colon as straight as possible while the rest of the intestines float down toward the diaphragm, away from the area being examined.

Some proctologists have hydraulic tables, which have a small ledge at the base. You kneel on the ledge, then rest your shoulder and your cheek on the table. One arm hangs down. This table provides greater support, allowing you to remain in the position longer. It also has floor pedals, similar to those on a dentist's chair. When a pedal is pressed, the table rises slightly. At the press of another pedal, the table tilts so that your head is tilted toward the floor.

NOW THAT YOU ARE READY . . .

The first thing you feel is the touch of the doctor's hands spreading your buttocks to see any clearly observable problems, such as a rash, external hemorrhoid, fissure, fistula, or prolapse. Next, the doctor inserts a gloved, lubricated finger into the anal opening and rests it there lightly, to give you a chance to get used to the touch and to relax the tight sphincter muscles that guard the entrance to the anal canal. Then the doctor inches the finger in very slowly, stretching the anal opening with gentle massage to make it a little wider. The doctor can feel the abutment of a woman's cervix or a man's prostate against the rectal wall and can also note any protrusions into the canal such as an enlarged prostate, tumors, abscesses, or foreign objects.

The doctor then withdraws the finger and inserts an anoscope, a three-inch tube with a light attached to it. Through the open end can be seen any abnormalities close to the anal opening, such as internal hemorrhoids, protruding papillae from the dentate line, or polyps in the lower third of the rectum.

If the doctor finds anything unusual or has reason to believe further investigation is necessary, he or she will either suggest an examination by a proctologist or gastroenterologist, or continue the examination with a sigmoidoscopy. Proctologists and gastroenterologists include a sigmoidoscopy in routine medical checkups.

The sigmoidoscopy, which requires considerable technical expertise, is as critical for diagnosis of early pathology as blood and urine tests, blood pressure measurements, Pap smears, and stool exams. The procedure is done with a sigmoidoscope, one of a group of instruments called endoscopes that are used to look through the entire gastrointestinal tract. Endoscopes inserted into the stomach are called gastroscopes; those inserted into the lower bowel a distance of no more than 25 inches are called sigmoidoscopes; and those inserted the full distance of the complete colon—75 inches—are called colonoscopes.

The Rectal Examination

For a sigmoidoscopy, you lie on your left side, parallel to the floor (rather than tilted on an angle). The doctor inserts the flexible fiberoptic sigmoidoscope into the rectal canal. This instrument is a 25-inch-long, rubberlike tube whose inner surface is lined with extremely thin, long glass fibers. These glass fibers are so optically correct that they transmit light along their entire length. Since both the rubber tube and the thin glass fibers are flexible, the doctor can guide the instrument around the intestine's many bends and loops. This instrument has completely replaced the old, rigid metal sigmoidoscope that is only 10 inches long. Newer instruments can transmit a digital image to a video screen.

Through the fiberoptic sigmoidoscope the doctor looks for polyps, cancerous growths, infection, and diverticuli (see Chapter 15) and takes great care to aim the instrument according to the bends and curves of the rectal canal and colon. The doctor moves the tube back and forth to bring all parts of the rectal and bowel wall into view. You may feel momentary cramping or discomfort when the instrument arrives at the top of the rectal canal, where the rectum joins the S-shaped sigmoid colon.

The doctor draws the instrument out very slowly in order to see any polyps along the way and observe the condition of the bowel lining. As the instrument presses along the valves of Houston, you may feel the desire to move your bowels, even though the enema or other preparation has already cleaned you out.

This marks the end of the routine proctological examination. The doctor wipes off any lubricant remaining on the anal opening and you are off the table and on your way, free from worry.

THE COLONOSCOPY

If sigmoidoscopy reveals any lesions, the next step is colonoscopy, performed primarily by proctologists or gastroenterologists. Often a rectal lesion signals the presence of a lesion higher up in the intestinal canal, within the range of the longer, 75-inch colonoscope. Like other endoscopes, the colonosocope has special attachments that can snip off tissue or cut off a growth with an electrified wire. The colonoscope can be guided all the way through the large intestine to the appendix and cecum where the small intestine ends.

During a routine physical checkup, former President Ronald Reagan had a sigmoidoscopy during which his doctor removed a rectal polyp. A year later, when a colonoscopy was done, a cancer was discovered higher up in the colon.

During the colonoscopic exam, you usually lie on your left side with your knees bent. Because of feelings of apprehension, the likelihood of some discomfort from cramping, and the length of time the procedure takes, the doctor will give you a tranquilizer and analgesic (painkiller).

THE BARIUM ENEMA X RAY

Not only has the fiberoptic sigmoidoscope replaced the 10-inch metal sigmoidoscope; it has also decreased use of the barium enema X ray, which was once used to delineate growths and other disorders in the colon all the way to the small intestine. Today, the colonoscope gives direct visualization of the entire colonic tract and enables the doctor to photograph the bowel lining. However, some doctors use the barium enema X ray as a confirmatory procedure that sometimes also reveals a lesion that the examiner missed. Sometimes, for technical reasons, the colonoscope cannot be advanced to the end of the intestine. The barium enema may help to visualize this area.

For this procedure, you will probably be referred to an X-ray specialist. You will be given an enema with a solution of barium sulfate, a metallic salt put into liquid form. This white suspension is impervious to X rays. As it floats up through the entire large intestine, an X ray shows how the column of barium liquid is shaped. Any uncommon dents or bulges may indicate a polyp, cancer, or ulcer.

You may feel some cramping during the barium enema because the solution presses against the colon wall. The enema and X ray take about 20 to 30 minutes, after which the barium is naturally expelled.

6

Constipation: The Major Cause of Hemorrhoids

■

Constipation is the difficult or infrequent passage of usually hard, dry stool. It is so uncomfortable that instead of waiting for the condition to pass or treating it, people often try to force defecation by pushing hard. Hemorrhoids result from the pressure.

Constipation is usually transient, such as when it coincides with emotional stress. Traumas such as divorce, the death of a loved one, or the loss of a job preoccupy the mind and put the bowels "on hold." Regularity usually resumes as emotions calm.

If one has a fissure, a rectal ulcer, or a painful hemorrhoid, defecation can cause additional pain. Delaying bowel movements causes constipation but spares the pain.

Constipation can also be a side effect of some tranquilizers, antacids, and other medications. Sometimes an alternative medication can be prescribed that will not have this effect.

Blockage of the bowel can also cause constipation. The bowel can sometimes be its own worst enemy. *Intussusception* (see Chapter 17) and *volvulus* (see Chapter 9) are two conditions in which the bowel blocks itself and prevents passage of feces.

For the most part, constipation is caused by consistently disregarding the gastrocolic reflex (the body's signal of readiness for a bowel movement) and by a poor diet lacking roughage and fluids, with excessive intake of meats, animal fats, and refined foods. *Learning to heed the gastrocolic reflex and improving the diet are the most important treatments of constipation.* To help you along upon occasion until bowel movements become regular again, you can use enemas, stool softeners, and, rarely if ever, laxatives.

ENEMAS

Among the three methods, enemas provide the most prompt relief and the least irritation. And they make the most sense physiologically: Why use a medication taken by mouth, which will affect the 30-foot lining of the intestinal tract, when an enema works faster and confines its effects to the specific area that needs loosening? Naturally, regular use of any of the methods makes you an "addict." As your intestines are deprived of the peristaltic exercise necessary for defecation, you lose the ability to initiate bowel movements.

A mild enema taken only occasionally, however, has no negative effects. The enema triggers movement of the bowel by stirring up and liquefying feces, churning them against the valves of Houston, and triggering the desire to defecate.

You can buy disposable plastic squeeze bottles containing a salt solution, or you can prepare your own at home. *Enemas should be a mixture of one tablespoon of salt to one quart of warm water.* This is called a physiologic salt solution, since it closely resembles the natural composition of the body's water content. Never omit the salt from the enema solution. Because of chemical reaction in the body called "osmotic pressure," large amounts of plain water should not be used because it can attract body salts through the membrane walls of the intestine; you will excrete them and lose a certain chemical balance. By the same token, using too much salt might cause the enema solution to pass through the membrane into the general system; this will also unbalance you chemically. Do not use cold water, as it might cause a spasm.

The saltwater solution is the only acceptable one. Never use soapsuds, and question any doctor who prescribes them, for they cause redness and irritation in the lining of the colon. One doctor chided a patient who used a soapsuds enema by telling him, "Don't put anything in an enema that you wouldn't put in your eye."

The old English term *turpentine stoop* referred to the use of that caustic substance in an enema. The lining would become so irritated and inflamed that the colon would go into a spasm. Naturally, therefore, the turpentine enema worked, but it did damage at the same time. Hot oil was another popular enema, until it also understandably fell out of favor.

Constipation can be so annoying and frustrating that people have used any type of enema, even harmful ones, to get relief. Yet the bowel responds just fine with the gentle salt solution, and any chemical or other additives are unnecessary and can even be damaging.

STOOL SOFTENERS

Hard, dry stool is difficult to pass. Stool softeners transform it into a soft, nonirritating stool that passes easily and does not create friction against hemorrhoids, fissures, or other anal disorders.

Stool softeners primarily consist of a bulk ingredient, such as cellulose. This forms a chemical sponge that both attracts and holds water, which is adsorbed to the outside of stool onto the molecules of stool softener. Colace, a stool softener, acts as a detergent that enables the stool to contain more water, thus increasing the stool's bulk.

Use a stool softener such as plain Colace or plain Dialose, avoiding any with added laxatives, which are harsh and irritating. A stool softener is usually able to get things moving by itself.

Stool softeners do not act as fast as enemas, since they must travel all the way from the mouth through the digestive tract to the large intestine. If the stool softener is in pill form, its gelatin capsule must dissolve before the softener can act.

LAXATIVES

When most people think of constipation, they immediately associate it with the word *laxative*. They may not even think of enemas or stool softeners as alternatives.

Yet laxatives have no place in your medicine cabinet. Years ago they were thought to be the best way to relieve constipation. Herbal laxatives such as senna leaf and oil of chenopodium were popular. Castor oil took over as a favorite, yet it is one of the strongest, most caustic laxatives in existence.

Later, chemically made laxatives were developed with advanced pharmacological techniques, particularly by the German school of chemistry. Chemists discovered that coal-tar derivatives had certain biological effects. Although some coal-tar products, such as aspirin, have been of great benefit in medical treatment, laxatives have been overused. They have created a following of people who are dependent on them for every bowel movement.

Laxatives should be used only as a last resort, with enemas or stool softeners taking precedence. If you use any laxative at all, choose milk of magnesia, which is the mildest and least irritating to your system. This should not be used often, however, by anyone with chronic kidney disease who may have difficulty excreting magnesium.

People whose doctors have recommended a salt-restricted diet should avoid laxatives containing sodium. Mineral oil is not recommended for several reasons. It interferes with the body's absorption of vitamins A, D, and E. It leaks from the rectum. And if given to infants, it may be inhaled into the lungs and lead to lipid pneumonia.

Neither laxatives nor enemas should ever be used if symptoms of appendicitis, such as fever or abdominal cramping, accompany constipation. Extreme peristalsis increases pressure within the intestinal tract and on the appendix, which may rupture. Individuals with colitis or diverticulitis should also be wary of causing this pressure.

Generally speaking, the only instance in which a laxative can be recommended is when the bowel must be cleaned out to allow a medical procedure such as the barium enema X ray or endoscopy.

7

Diarrhea: The Traveler's Route to Hemorrhoids

■

Janet had never had a hint of hemorrhoids in her life. But after a month vacationing in South America, she found she had brought them home as an unwelcome souvenir. Although the foreign food had been delicious and the water cold and sparkling, to her digestive tract they were alien substances containing unfamiliar bacteria and parasites that had to be rejected. The result: diarrhea, the body's way of throwing off offending substances. Diarrhea is a twofold increase in frequency of unformed bowel movement accompanied by cramping or nausea, urgency, chills, fever, or malaise. Hemorrhoids can develop from the expulsive force of loose, watery stool.

Of course diarrhea can afflict armchair travelers as well as those who rack up frequent-flyer miles. Many people have experienced diarrhea. It can be frightening and very uncomfortable. But diarrhea is usually not a serious health threat unless it lasts more than two days, occurs along with other illnesses, or develops in infants or very young children who run the immediate risk of dehydration. Extreme loss of fluids can also sometimes create a state of shock.

Diarrhea can be caused by allergic reactions to milk or other food, stress or anxiety, an adverse reaction to purgatives (harsh laxatives such as castor oil or croton oil), and certain antibiotics. Contaminated food may be the biggest culprit. Each year, an estimated 5 million people become ill in the United States from foodborne diseases, and 5,000 die.

TRAVELER'S DIARRHEA

As the global village has gotten smaller over the years, with planes busily crisscrossing the earth and people vacationing in remote, intriguing spots, *traveler's diarrhea* has attracted increasing attention. Traveler's diarrhea usually consists of four to five loose bowel movements per day and lasts three to four days. Persistent diarrhea is uncommon; chronic diarrhea must be diagnosed to be properly treated.

Travelers get diarrhea from ingesting contaminated food or water. Especially risky foods are raw meat and seafood, and raw fruit and vegetables. Tap water, ice, and unpasteurized milk and dairy products are also dangerous. Safe beverages include bottled carbonated (especially flavored) drinks, beer, wine, hot coffee and tea, and water that is boiled or treated with chlorine or iodine.

Many bacteria cause traveler's diarrhea. The most common is *Escherichia coli bacillus*, while *Salmonella* and *Campylobacter* (and, less commonly, *Shigella*) cause outbreaks of food-associated diarrhea throughout the industrialized world. The *Vibrio bacillus* associated with the ingestion of raw or poorly cooked seafood has been known to cause diarrhea in passengers on tropical cruise ships. Although parasites like *Giardia, Entamoeba*, and tapeworm are not major causes of acute diarrhea, they should not be ruled out in persisting, unexplained cases.

A TRAVELER'S ADVISORY

The risk of contracting traveler's diarrhea is greater in the developing countries of Latin America, Africa, the Middle East, and Asia. Lower risk areas are Canada, the United States, Australia, New Zealand, and some Caribbean islands. Although northern Europe is also a low-risk area, bacillary dysentery and typhoid are common in southern Europe during the summer and autumn.

Foodborne and waterborne diseases such as those caused by amoeba and bacilli are common throughout central and tropical South America. In the temperate part of South America, such as in Argentina, Chile, and Uruguay, salmonella infection is common. Parasitic infection is widespread. In Asia, contaminated food and water are a common cause of diarrheal disease and hepatitis.

PREVENTING AND TREATING DIARRHEA

The surest way to prevent diarrhea is to pay meticulous attention to food and beverage preparation. Travelers to foreign lands are often required to be inoculated against a variety of diseases, but there is no effective vaccine against traveler's diarrhea. Antiperistaltic agents such as diphenoxylate and atropine (marketed as Lomotil) and loperamide (marketed as Imodium) are not preventive. Bismuth subsalicylate (marketed as Pepto-Bismol) decreases the incidence of diarrhea, but in large doses may be harmful, especially to individuals currently taking aspirin. Two antimicrobial medicines, doxycycline and TMP-SMX (a sulfa derivative), are said to reduce the chance of getting traveler's diarrhea and to treat diarrhea associated with nausea, vomiting, high fever, and bloody stools, but are not currently recommended for preventive use because of potential side effects.

Antidiarrheal medications can ease the severity of spasm and diminish both the number of bowel movements and the quantity eliminated. Medications that adsorb toxins give stools more consistency but do not decrease the cramps or diarrhea. Therefore only partial relief can be gained from the most commonly used adsorbents: pectin (better known as a thickener of jams and jellies) and kaolin (derived from the fine, thirsty clay used to produce translucent quality in Chinese pottery and Limoges china). To reduce the "clenched fist" of diarrheal spasm, some medications also contain paregoric (tincture of opium). Attapulgite (marketed as Kaopectate), which can be bought over-the-counter, effectively adsorbs bacteria and some parasites, enabling the body to eliminate them.

Bismuth salicylate (Pepto-Bismol) decreases the frequency of defecation by one-half but may be toxic if taken by a person with kidney disease or intolerance of salicylates.

Antimotility agents (opiates such as paregoric and codeine) or loperamide (Imodium) provide temporary relief of cramping but should not be used by anyone with high fever or blood in stools.

People who have glaucoma should not use medication containing belladonna or atropine. Scopolamine, a sedative, is of dubious value. Lactobacillus culture (found in yogurt) may help to restore the normal balance of bacteria in the colonic tract if the diarrhea is caused by a reaction to antibiotics.

Always consult a physician if diarrhea persists longer than three or four days or occurs along with high fever, blood and mucus in stool, severe cramping, or dehydration. But if diarrhea has a rapid onset and lasts for less than two days, you can probably treat it yourself.

Most often, treatment for diarrhea consists of waiting it out. It is important to drink plenty of potable water, clear soup, and fruit juices, and to eat salted crackers to replace water and salts lost during diarrhea. Eating rice or bananas can make diarrhea less debilitating. Avoid roughage such as bran and raw vegetables, red meat, milk and other dairy products, and coffee and colas that contain caffeine.

8

For the Pregnant Woman

∎

Elaine had heard of a craving for pickles and ice cream during pregnancy but did not expect this sudden desire for mixed nuts. Yet one afternoon she ate more than half a pound of them, got diarrhea, and developed hemorrhoids that stayed until the baby was born.

Hemorrhoids are often a problem during pregnancy, when the growing fetus places pressure on hemorrhoidal blood vessels, causing rectal veins to distend. Intense pushing during labor might also create hemorrhoids. So does constipation, which usually results from insufficient roughage, inadequate exercise, and pressure of the fetus on the intestines.

By obeying the gastrocolic reflex, eating properly, and getting daily exercise, a woman can often prevent constipation and keep hemorrhoids from forming or from becoming a major problem.

Many women find that eating small, frequent meals

rather than three large ones aids digestion and elimination during pregnancy. It is important to eat raw vegetables and fruits and bran daily for roughage, and to drink plenty of fluids to keep stool soft and easy to pass. Avoid laxatives and other orally ingested treatment for constipation, as well as all medications that could affect the fetus. Prune juice, prunes, figs, and other dried fruits act as natural laxatives and provide iron, an essential nutrient.

Some women become very fatigued during pregnancy and exercise less. Join a prenatal exercise class to improve body tone and to strengthen muscles you will use during childbirth.

Fortunately, *hemorrhoids that develop during pregnancy usually disappear by themselves several weeks after childbirth*. Therefore, surgery and other treatments requiring an anesthetic are not recommended. Prevent irritation to hemorrhoids by inserting petroleum jelly inside the anal canal with your finger before and between bowel movements. Warm sitz baths can also help but are often not recommended during the final months of pregnancy, as water can seep into the vagina. Try applying hot towels to the anus to reduce swelling and spasm of sphincter muscles. Use ice packs if there is some bleeding. Consult your doctor about the advisability of an analgesic ointment, such as a "-caine" derivative, if hemorrhoids are painful.

9

Special Problems of the Elderly

■

Hemorrhoids resulting from chronic constipation are so common among the elderly that one 83-year-old woman flatly stated that she wondered whether anyone her age did not suffer from them.

"It's a constant cry among my friends," she said. "But at this state of the game it's an accepted thing. We don't function as regularly as in earlier years; our teeth are either bad or false, so we don't eat much fruit or roughage. And our nerves are shattered by all the things we have to cope with. I'm sure that has an effect on stomach function."

Look in the refrigerators of many elderly people, and you will see bland foods that are easy to chew: applesauce, eggs, soup, boiled chicken, processed cheese. In the medicine cabinet: several brands of laxatives, glycerin suppositories, an anesthetic ointment or two. Their diet includes little roughage, so their stools are hard and dry. Age weakens abdominal and sphincter muscles, diminishing their ability to pass a hard, dry stool. The laxative habit among the elderly is common; many people begin relying on laxatives in middle age, after years of poor diet and faulty bowel habits. By the time citizens are truly senior, they may have sampled every product in the drugstore and swear they cannot have a bowel movement without the aid of a laxative.

Consider the thousands of physically inactive or bedridden elderly people who live in nursing homes. If they are confined to a bed or a wheelchair, they get no exercise at all and may rely for every bowel movement on laxatives and enemas given by nurses.

Constipation is a difficult problem for the elderly who have become so dependent on laxatives that they just cannot "kick the habit." They should try using stool softeners to ease the passage of stool, and plain petroleum jelly inserted into the anal canal to minimize irritation. This is much more effective than suppositories, which have many elderly devotees. Yet suppositories are often ineffective. They can slide so far up in the rectum that their effect is lost on the anal canal, which needs lubrication most. A weekly enema of saline solution, one tablespoon of salt in a quart of warm water, can often be the best help of all.

Chronic constipation frequently brings on hemorrhoids and keeps them painful and inflamed. Elderly persons usually have combined internal and external hemorrhoids. Sometimes internal ones can be caused by an enlarged prostate stretching the mucosa of the anorectal canal. Hemorrhoids can be relieved by self-care methods such as warm sitz baths, use of a lubricant and/or anesthetic ointment if hemorrhoids are painful, stool softeners, and change of diet.

Special Problems of the Elderly

Fecal impaction may be another result of constipation. A hard, dry stool may not pass from the body but lodges in the rectum and obstructs all further elimination, sometimes causing abdominal cramping and distension. The stool must be broken into smaller pieces with the finger and pulled out of the anal canal.

Sometimes the opposite problem occurs. Anal sphincter muscles can become so weak and flaccid that one may lose the capacity to control the bowels, suffering the humiliation of feces leaking onto underclothing or the bed. The only recourse is to use the toilet every hour or so to reduce the chance of leakage.

Some elderly people live in a confused, disoriented state of mental isolation, as though they are living in their own private world. They may not even be aware of their own incontinence. If they live in a nursing home, they may be diapered; if the nursing home staff tends not to clean them up after every incontinence, they can suffer irritated and chafed skin and ulcers in addition to their other problems.

Weakened anal sphincter muscles can allow the rectal lining or the entire anal wall thickness to slide outside the anal opening, a condition called prolapse (lining only) or procidentia (complete wall thickness). To hold these structures in place, a silver wire is inserted under the skin, encircling the narrowed anal opening like a drawstring.

Any change in usual bowel function—such as sudden constipation or diarrhea, ineffectual desire to move bowels with passage of only gas, or discharge of blood or mucus— necessitates complete examination of the colonic tract by a proctologist or gastroenterologist.

VOLVULUS

Volvulus is derived from the Latin word *volvo*, meaning to wind, turn, roll, or twist around. This condition occurs when a segment of bowel twists on its long axis, much as an oblong balloon can be twisted so that it appears cinched at the center. Volvulus is more common in the elderly but may occur in the newborn. The symptoms and treatment are identical to those for intussusception (see Chapter 17).

IT'S NEVER TOO LATE TO IMPROVE BOWEL HABITS

Advancing age makes eating a proper diet—including bran, raw fruits and vegetables, and plenty of water and other fluids—even more important. Prune juice can help soften the stool and stimulate the peristalsis necessary for defecation. Even when it is not possible to chew raw fruits and vegetables, stirring some bran into applesauce is one way to add roughage to your diet. This may not allow the laxative-dependent person to "de-lax," but it may cut down on the frequency of taking laxatives.

If you are able, try to include some exercise in your daily routine, such as walking or swimming. And try this exercise to specifically strengthen the abdominal muscles, improve bowel movements, and help you avoid constipation: Lie on your back and slowly draw one knee and then the other up to your chest. It is a relaxing exercise that you may come to look forward to doing every day.

10

Self-Care of Hemorrhoids

■

The presence of hemorrhoids does not necessarily require medical treatment—though you must make sure the problem is really hemorrhoids and not something more serious (see Chapter 4). Make sure you have a rectal examination by a proctologist or gastroenterologist to confirm that hemorrhoids alone are causing your symptoms.

If hemorrhoids do not cause real discomfort, they should be left alone.

The most important steps in treating hemorrhoids and constipation are identical to the ways used to prevent them:

- Heed the "call of nature" and allow time for bowel movements after both breakfast and dinner.
- Include roughage in your diet.
- Drink plenty of water and other fluids.
- Exercise to promote good muscle tone.
- Avoid pushing too hard or too long during bowel movements.

View all these practices as long-range and permanent changes in your approach to health care. But until they provide permanent relief from hemorrhoids, you can take some more immediate measures to get temporary relief from discomfort or pain.

THE SITZ BATH

Take a 15-minute bath several times a day, after bowel movements if possible, to relieve hemorrhoids by reducing swelling and easing spasms of anal sphincter muscles. The bath water should be hot but not burning hot. Do not add anything to the bath water such as bubble bath, Epsom salts, bath oil, or even soap. These can irritate swollen hemorrhoids. The sitz bath will soothe you—and even let you catch up on reading.

THE KNEE-CHEST POSITION

The knee-chest position relieves the pull of gravity on rectal veins. Kneel on the floor and rest on your left shoulder and the left side of your face, with buttocks lifted in the air. Breathe slowly and deeply. Staying in this position for even a few minutes is beneficial. Some people even read while in this position for a half hour or so.

WIPE GENTLY

Wiping too hard with toilet paper can badly irritate hemorrhoids and cause bleeding. Try using moistened cotton balls or rinsing with water after a bowel movement. Pat dry.

STOOL SOFTENERS AND LUBRICATION

When hard, dry stool passes from the body, it may irritate hemorrhoids and cause bleeding. A stool softener (not a laxative) softens the stool by making it adsorb more liquid. This stool is easier to pass and creates less friction on hemorrhoids. (For more information on stool softeners, see Chapter 6.)

Another way to reduce friction from stool passage is to lubricate the anal canal. Insert plain petroleum jelly or another lubricant such as K-Y Jelly with your finger, making sure the lubricant is actually inside the anal canal, not just outside on the anal opening. Then wash your hands thoroughly to prevent accidental transmission of anal bacteria.

OVER-THE-COUNTER PREPARATIONS FOR HEMORRHOID RELIEF

A medical truism is that if there are many claimed cures for an illness, there is no real cure. Over the ages, countless formulas have been devised for treating hemorrhoids. They have ranged from pastes of slippery elm powder or other herbal remedies, to the application of leeches, lead, mercury, bismuth, and coal tar. Some of these probably caused more bleeding and infections than they prevented. Honey, cloves, and ground-up shells and bones have found their way into many home remedies. Some people swear by the use of a garlic clove as a suppository, though garlic is certainly not an ingredient in any ointment or salve now on the market. Some ingredients that are listed, however, are just as questionable, and some are even dangerous.

The basic ingredient in any hemorrhoid medication is a lubricant to ease friction and irritation. Modern hemorrhoid remedies contain cod-liver oil, vegetable oil, cocoa butter, lanolin, glycerin, petrolatum, and, most peculiarly, shark-liver oil. Plain petroleum jelly inserted into the anal canal with a finger is just as effective as any of these—and cheaper.

Some manufacturers add ingredients to the basic lubricant to give more potent "temporary relief." Anesthetic agents that slightly deaden pain nerves are usually "-caine" derivatives, such as benzocaine or lidocaine. An ointment containing an anesthetic is likely to give a measure of added relief, but it may also cause an allergic reaction. Taking a hot sitz bath is less convenient than using an ointment, but it does give temporary relief with no side effects.

Manufacturers may also add astringents—such as tannic acid, bismuth or zinc compounds, belladonna compounds, ephedrine, and phenylephrine—and claim that these reduce swelling by constricting capillaries. But hemorrhoids are not capillaries. They are veins, and astringents have no effect on them. They may only reduce secondary swelling around them.

Vitamins A and D and yeast-cell extracts are added to promote healing of irritated tissues, but there is little or no evidence that they have this effect.

Other relatively useless ingredients are antiseptics such as boric acid, menthol, resorcinol, and mercury compound. Although they may have a slight effect on bacteria or parasites, the concentrations in which they appear in the lubricant base render them ineffective.

All these ingredients appear in various combinations at the drugstore, packaged as ointments, creams, suppositories, or sprays. Each manufacturer privately determines how many of these ingredients to add to the basic lubricant.

Ointments and creams, since they are applied with the fingers, lubricate more effectively than other preparation forms. Some, however, come with a plastic nozzle that is to be inserted into the anal canal. If the nozzle is not inserted properly, the canal can be traumatized. Fingers are safer.

Suppositories are easy to insert, but can slide up high in the rectal canal. After they melt, their effect on low-lying hemorrhoidal veins is delayed or lost completely. Aerosol sprays are convenient but hard to use accurately, which makes them useless as well. Aerosol sprays also contain gases that may be harmful to the environment. Applying lubricants with the finger may not be as fastidious as using suppositories or sprays, but it does get the medication in the right place, at the right time, in the right quantity.

THIS OINTMENT MAY BE HAZARDOUS TO YOUR HEALTH

Some ingredients in hemorrhoid remedies can be dangerous. Belladonna and atropine can cause urinary retention in some men with enlarged prostates. They can also bring on an acute attack of glaucoma in susceptible people. Ephedrine increases blood pressure and must be avoided by hypertensive people. Some people may also have allergic reactions to "-caine" derivatives.

DON'T PAY FOR THE HYPE

Hemorrhoids cannot be improved with medication, which may even be harmful to some people. Long-term relief comes from improving bowel habits by heeding the "call of nature," adding roughage to your diet, and other methods described in Chapter 12. For relief of pain, you might apply anesthetic agents such as "-caine" derivatives once or twice, only if you have no known history of allergy to Novocain or other "-caine" drugs. If pain continues, obtain temporary relief from sitz baths, acetaminophen, stool softeners, and lubricating with petroleum jelly until you can see your doctor.

Never treat rectal bleeding with over-the-counter medications. For the most part, they do not stop bleeding. More important, bleeding may be a sign of cancer and must be checked by a physician.

Rectal itching, however, can often benefit by the use of cortisone ointment for short periods only. Even though some cortisone ointments are sold over-the-counter, it is still better to consult a physician about their use.

11

How a Doctor Treats Hemorrhoids

■

AILMENTS OVER THE CENTURIES

Forever, it seems, people have suffered from anal and rectal problems. A description of rectal prolapse appears in the second book of Chronicles in the Bible: "And it came to pass, that in process of time, after the end of two years, his bowels fell out by reason of his sickness: so he died of sore diseases." In Deuteronomy and Samuel, Ashbod was "smitten with emerods," meaning hemorrhoids. The Egyptians and Hindus both recorded clinical information on hemorrhoids and fistulas. In the ruins of Pompeii, a bronze *speculum ani*, quite similar to today's anoscope, was found amid shards of pottery and human bones.

Hippocrates, born in 460 B.C., developed methods of treating hemorrhoids and fistulas that continue to be used today. Celsus, a doctor at the time of Augustus and Tiberius, became famous for his treatment of fistulas and was nicknamed the Latin Hippocrates. Paulus Aegineta, who published *The Treatise of Surgery* about A.D. 600, has also been compared to Hippocrates.

The history of medicine is filled with ironic and tragic stories. During the reign of Henry Plantagenet in fourteenth-century England, a surgeon named John of Arderne invented an operation for the cure of fistulas. Yet only a century later, Henry V died at the age of 35 from a badly infected fistula, for Arderne's teachings had been lost. They were not rediscovered until 500 years later.

The French have long been fashion trendsetters, but in 1686 some went too far in their desire to be *au courant*. When Louis XIV developed a fistula, members of his court asserted that they, too, were afflicted with a "point of honor," and some even had unnecessary surgery. The court surgeon, Dr. M. Faelix, used a sickle-shaped knife, later called the Bistouri Royal.

The leader of modern proctology was Dr. Frederick Salmon, founder in 1835 of St. Mark's Hospital in London, which became the center of proctological research and inventiveness. Most proctologists today follow Dr. Salmon's methods.

THE RECALCITRANT HEMORRHOID

When a hemorrhoid is inordinately painful or large, or bleeds profusely, self-care methods are often ineffective or provide only temporary relief.

Doctors use six methods to treat hemorrhoids: injection, banding, freezing, laser, electric current, and surgery. The first three can be used only with internal hemorrhoids, because the pain nerves in the skin covering external hemorrhoids make the methods too painful to endure without an anesthetic. However, if a person has both internal and external hemorrhoids, treatment of internal ones often relieves external ones as well.

The Injection Method

The injection method involves injecting an internal hemorrhoid with phenol in oil or quinine in urea. The liquid glues the vein walls to each other, collapsing and shrinking the vein. If the shrunken vein is no longer subjected to excess pressure, the hemorrhoid disappears.

The Banding Method

The banding method is a direct descendant of Hippocrates' method of tying a thread around an internal hemorrhoid, cutting off blood flow and eventually causing the hemorrhoid to fall off. Today, a doctor pushes a special rubber band, more tensile than a thread, onto the base of the hemorrhoid with an applicator. The band acts like a tourniquet to cut off the blood supply. About a week later, the dried-up hemorrhoid shrinks and falls off along with the band. Banding is a minor procedure that rarely necessitates losing time from work. It is not painful, but some people feel a dull ache until the hemorrhoid falls off.

The Freezing Method

The freezing method is also known as cryosurgery. The cryosurgery apparatus reduces liquid nitrogen or nitrous oxide to a subfreezing temperature, as low as 80 degrees below zero. A frozen applicator tip touched to the hemorrhoid freezes it into a "vein popsicle." During the next two or three weeks, the frozen hemorrhoid melts, shrinks, and eventually falls off.

As it melts, moisture around the anal opening must be absorbed by a pad, such as a sanitary napkin or a folded towel held in place by a napkin belt, a T-binder (similar to an athletic supporter), or snug-fitting underwear. Most of the drainage occurs during the first few days after the cryosurgery. For the next couple of weeks, drainage steadily decreases. The drainage may create an odor, but usually the only discomfort is a throbbing or tingling sensation. Most people continue normal activity after undergoing the procedure.

At one time cryosurgery was popular, but it has largely fallen into disuse.

The Laser Method

Laser is an acronym for Light Amplification by Stimulating the Emission of Radiation. Laser can be compared to the rapid transmittal of electrons along an insulated wire to cause intense heat at its tip. This heat-producing system is used in toasters and electric ovens, and in electric cautery instruments to coagulate and destroy tissue. Laser is different in that it uses rapidly moving light waves instead of electrons.

Laser instruments issue light waves so rapidly that tissue absorbs their energy as heat. The tips of laser instruments are made of synthetic sapphire or garnet and use substances such as carbon dioxide, argon, or ND-YAG (neodynium-ytrium, aluminum, garnet) to amplify the light waves' motion by emitting radiation.

The laser method coagulates the hemorrhoid into a dry, shrunken, raisinlike stubble. This procedure is an improvement over electrocautery or cryotherapy because it provides better control over the depth of coagulation and the amount of bleeding, and reduces postoperative oozing and discomfort. Regular activities can be resumed within a week. Laser hemorrhoidectomy can usually be done as an ambulatory procedure with no hospitalization.

Electric current

Electric current is the newest of all the techniques. Either direct or alternating current is used to transmit enough energy to the tip of a probe to coagulate a hemorrhoid. The activated probe lightly touches the hemorrhoid, and the transmitted electrical energy causes the tissue to blanch as a sizzling noise is heard. The hemorrhoid, now coagulated, starts to shrink. This painless procedure is performed in the doctor's office. The electric current technique appears to be highly effective, but it needs more clinical trials before it is established as an accepted treatment for hemorrhoids.

Surgery

Many doctors opt for the preceding methods over surgery because recovery is quicker and they cost less. Other doctors, however, nearly always prefer surgery because expertly performed surgery results in a minimum of bleeding and stenosis, the formation of scar tissue that may obstruct the anal opening. Ask your doctor about the pros and cons of the different treatments. If you are unsure which to choose, get a second opinion.

The preferred method today is probably laser therapy, but surgery is often recommended if an internal hemorrhoid is particularly large and troublesome, or if an external hemorrhoid is large, painful, bleeding, or causes excruciating itching. Surgical hemorrhoidectomy requires an anesthetic and hospitalization for five to seven days. The surgeon cuts off the hemorrhoid and closes the cut with absorbable stitches that do not have to be removed. Doctors usually prescribe painkillers for the first few days after the operation and recommend bedrest at home for a week to 10 days after discharge from the hospital. A small anal pad placed on the anal opening catches any drainage. It is kept in place simply by the buttock muscles, snug-fitting underwear, or a T-binder. There is far less drainage after a hemorrhoidectomy than after other methods.

Very warm sitz baths twice a day and after bowel movements are soothing. Add nothing to the water—no soap, disinfectant, or Epsom salts. See your doctor weekly for the six to eight weeks after surgery so any signs of infection can be diagnosed and treated early. Then resume normal activity, but for another month or so avoid strenuous activities such as heavy lifting and jogging.

12

How to Prevent Hemorrhoids

■

Imagine a tribesman who lives in conditions we would call primitive. Every day he hunts game, but he also gets much of his food from the plant kingdom, eating it raw. His hunting gives him plenty of exercise, and his diet contains a good amount of roughage. But it is a third factor that makes it especially unlikely that he will ever experience hemorrhoids, constipation, or other problems that vex "civilized" society. Every morning and evening after he has eaten, the tribesman knows that his body will automatically signal readiness for a bowel movement. He waits for the signal before he goes off to hunt. He knows that after a bowel movement he will be more physiologically responsive to his environment: lighter, more relaxed, and alert.

Compare his daily regimen with that of a businessman in today's industrialized society. He breakfasts on coffee and a sweet roll—no roughage there. Immediately after swallowing the last drop of coffee, he grabs his briefcase, rushes out to the car, and drives to work. He has a feeling of needing to have a bowel movement, but he is in too much of a hurry.

Once at the office, he gets so caught up with hunting down solutions to problems that he ignores the feeling of wanting to defecate. There is no time to waste going to the bathroom. Eventually the urge subsides.

For lunch he has a hamburger and soft drink delivered and eats hurriedly at his desk. After work he considers going to the gym to work out, but as usual he is too tired. He drives home. Dinner is lamb chops, French fries, canned peas, coffee, and chocolate cake. Now, he thinks, there is finally time for the bowel movement he has postponed all day. He sits on the toilet, reads a magazine, and waits for something to happen. But just because he is finally ready does not mean his bowels will cooperate. They have their own natural timetable, which he has ignored. He pushes and strains, aggravating hemorrhoids he has had for a while.

He decides to take a laxative. It causes such an explosive bowel movement that his hemorrhoids are more irritated than before. He curses and smoothes on a widely advertised ointment that claims to reduce hemorrhoidal pain and swelling. The ointment feels nice, but if truth be told, it does not really help any more than plain (and less expensive) petroleum jelly would.

By ignoring the urge to defecate in the morning, eating a diet of fatty and processed foods, and failing to exercise, this man counts himself as one of the millions of people for whom hemorrhoids and constipation are a way of life. He needs to learn that the conditions' prevention and cure are largely the same: improving bowel habits by heeding the "call of nature," eating a healthier diet, and getting enough exercise.

THE "CALL OF NATURE"

The "call of nature" is not Tarzan's cry or the yearning to explore wilderness. It is another term for the gastrocolic reflex, which signals the body's readiness for a bowel movement. The reflex nearly always occurs in the morning and evening and is triggered by eating and drinking. The digestive tract receives new food to digest and is ready to release what has already been digested and transformed into waste. Feces travel through the large intestine to the rectum, where they rest on the shelflike valves of Houston. The feces' weight causes the valves' nerves to transmit to the brain the signal that it is time for a bowel movement. If a person obeys this signal consistently, a regular elimination schedule naturally results.

The gastrocolic reflex is so fundamental to normal body functioning that obeying it should feel as natural and inevitable as eating when you are hungry, drinking when you are thirsty, and sleeping when you are tired. Yet many people deprive themselves of the reflex's benefits. Instead of allowing themselves to respond to the reflex, they rush off to school or work after breakfast, or to a meeting or a movie after dinner—the very times the reflex is most likely to occur. Or some people dislike the act of defecating and avoid it as long as possible. People who live in crowded households with inadequate bathroom facilities may be forced to postpone defecation in deference to logistical problems.

Time allowed for a bowel movement after both breakfast and dinner is time well spent. It can both prevent and relieve constipation and the pushing and straining that can cause hemorrhoids. Of course, "regularity" differs among individuals. Not everyone naturally has two bowel movements daily; normal frequency for one person may be three times a day, and for someone else, only once every two days. The important thing is to heed your body's signals, and the best way to start is by mentally "listening" for them after breakfast and dinner.

A HEALTHIER DIET FOR HEALTHIER BOWELS

The typical American diet is believed to contribute to constipation, hemorrhoids, colon-rectal cancer, and other bowel problems. Refined, processed foods with little fiber content and meats and animal fats in large quantities contribute to bowel malfunction and disease. These foods do not provide the bulk and roughage the intestines need to form an easily passed stool and to stimulate the peristaltic action that keeps feces moving through the intestinal tract.

Add bulk and roughage to the diet by eating raw vegetables and fruits, and bran and other whole grains. Bran is especially useful because it absorbs many times its weight in water, making the stool soft, moist, and easier to pass. Packaged bran cereals, preferably those with little or no added sugar and additive-free, can be a significant addition to the diet. Unprocessed bran (sometimes called miller's bran, since in grain mills it is removed along with wheat germ to make refined white flour) has a coarse texture, but it becomes quite soft and usually unnoticeable when combined with other foods.

Drink plenty of water. This aids elimination by keeping stools soft. People on weight-loss diets that call for eight glasses of water per day have often been pleasantly surprised by the resulting improvement in bowel movements. Fruit and vegetable juices are also good to drink, though they add calories. Coffee can be irritating, especially to people with a sensitive stomach. Anyone troubled by excess gas should not drink carbonated soft drinks, which themselves contain gas.

It may take some time for your system to get used to roughage if it has been notably lacking in your diet. To avoid excess gas or abdominal discomfort, alter your diet gradually, over a period of several weeks. Start by eating a bran cereal for breakfast. After you have eaten more roughage for a month or so, you will probably wonder how you ever managed without it. If excessive flatulence still occurs, consult Chapter 13 for diet tips.

HOW TO GET HEALTHY BOWELS THROUGH DIET

Every day:
- Eat plenty of raw vegetables and fruits.
- Drink plenty of water and other fluids.
- Include bran in your diet.
- Reduce your intake of meats, animal fats, alcoholic beverages, and chemical additives.

Easy Ways to Improve Your Diet

Instead of . . .	Substitute . . .
Low-fiber breakfast cereals	Bran cereals, oatmeal, Wheatena; *or* add unprocessed bran to regular breakfast cereals
Sugar on cereal	Raisins, currants, chopped dates, or other dried fruits on cold or hot cereals
Meat, animal fats, chemical additives and preservatives	Fish, whole grains, dried peas and beans, chicken in moderation, polyunsaturated oils
Overcooked or canned vegetables	Raw vegetables salads and very lightly steamed spinach and other fresh greens and vegetables
Canned sweetened fruit	Raw fresh fruit
White bread	Whole-grain bread, bran muffins, corn bread (made with stone-ground cornmeal); *or* add a couple of tablespoons of bran and wheat germ to home-baked goods
White rice	Brown rice, kasha (buckwheat groats), bulgur wheat, other whole grains
White-flour cakes and cookies, puddings	Whole-wheat cakes and cookies, *or* white flour with bran added; fresh fruit salad; prune compote (cook prunes, dried apricots, and lemon wedges in water five to 10 minutes)
TV snacks of potato chips, cookies, low-fiber crackers, processed cheese, candy	Raw carrots, celery, cucumber, sweet pepper sticks, plain or with yogurt dip (try yogurt and blue cheese)
Soft drinks, coffee	Water, fruit and vegetable juices

> **SMART WAYS TO INCLUDE BRAN IN YOUR DIET**
>
> In addition to eating a bran cereal for breakfast, take unprocessed bran in milk, juice, or coffee; or "hide" bran in soups, gravies, spaghetti and other sauces, chili, stew, casseroles, batter for fried chicken, dips, peanut butter, tuna and egg salads, salad dressing, sandwich spreads, meat loaf, pancakes, French toast batter, crumb topping, and baked goods.

THE IMPORTANCE OF EXERCISE

People with good muscle tone are less likely to develop hemorrhoids than people who allow their muscles to become lax and flabby. Yoga, running, dancing, walking, swimming, aerobics, and other forms of exercise strengthen the body, including those muscles used in effective, normal defecation: abdominal, gluteal (buttocks), and sphincter muscles.

An incidental benefit of exercise is that it makes you thirsty, so you naturally drink more water. Also, contrary to popular belief, exercise makes you less hungry, not more. It also improves metabolism and digestion.

One exercise may specifically strengthen the anal sphincter muscles. The "buttock press" involves rhythmically tightening and relaxing the buttock muscles. As the buttocks press together, you should be able to feel the anal sphincter muscles tighten, too. This exercise is analogous to the "Kegel" exercises many women use to strengthen vaginal muscles.

The buttock press is so easy and unobtrusive that it can be done several times a day—while sitting at a desk, waiting for a bus, riding in an elevator, or washing dishes. It is an especially valuable exercise for pregnant women, and for the elderly, the bedridden, and other people who do not get enough exercise.

EASY GOING

Normal bowel movements do not require straining and forcing, which often result in pushing out rectal veins, which swell into hemorrhoids. If defecation is sometimes difficult, do not strain. Wait for a while, then try again.

When you are on the toilet, be aware of how your body feels. Many people read on the toilet, since it may be the only place they can find peace and quiet! Reading for short periods of time is probably fine. But reading may make you insensitive to how forcefully and long you might be pushing.

13

Flatulence

The act of expelling gas anally is called flatulence. The gas itself is called flatus. While flatulence is not really a disorder—a certain amount of flatus is produced every day as a natural result of digestion—too much, especially if it is uncontrollable, can be a problem.

The act of uncontrolled passage of gas is very embarrassing, especially when it is loud and the gas is foul-smelling, and is obnoxious to people nearby. During the Roman Empire, laws were passed penalizing people who passed gas in public places. The English explorer Richard Burton told of a certain African tribe whose members, while sitting around a council fire, would emphasize their pontifications by passing wind at the appropriate moments. At the Moulin Rouge in Paris, at the turn of this century, the entertainer Joseph Puzol (called Le Petomane) performed by passing gas in a manner that reproduced the tunes of popular songs. This unique talent entitled him to be known as the "father of flatology."

The ability to steadily contain flatus depends on muscles that are part of the anal wall itself—the internal anal sphincter. Outside, but around the anal canal wall, is another set of muscles called the external sphincters. These muscles control, on demand, the forceful expulsion of gas. When these two sets of muscles, the internal and external sphincters, do not react synchronously, uncontrollable flatulence occurs.

Flatus mostly contains five different gases:

Oxygen and *nitrogen* are derived from swallowed air. Part of these gases are absorbed by the lining of the gut, and the rest emerge as flatus.

Carbon dioxide is created from the action of stomach acids on food, or by the action of bacteria in the colon on unabsorbed sugar.

Hydrogen is produced mostly by the action of colon bacteria on unabsorbed sugar.

Methane is unrelated to food intake. Only about 30 percent of the population produces methane; of these, the maximum amount is first produced at about eight years of age, and the amount continues unchanged throughout life. The buoyancy of stool is mostly due to methane, not to fat.

All five of these gases are odorless. The offensive smell of flatus is caused primarily by infinitesimal, trace amounts of hydrogen sulfide, ammonia, mercaptan, indole, and skatole. These are by-products of the digestive process.

ORDINARY SUGARS:
NOT SO SIMPLE TO DIGEST

Sugar ingestion plays a major role in gas production. The word *sugar* is the catch-all, generic term for different types of related, often sweet compounds. There are simple sugars (glucose, fructose, galactose), and there are complex sugars (such as sucrose and lactose) composed of different simple sugars of varying types bound together by chemical linkages. The site for the absorption of sugars is the small intestine. Here simple sugars are readily absorbed. Complex sugars cannot always be completely absorbed because their component simple sugars have resistant linkages. Therefore some complex sugars pass along the gut to the large intestine, where resident bacteria act on them and gas (mostly hydrogen and carbon dioxide) forms.

Ordinary table sugar (sucrose) is a complex sugar in that it consists of glucose bound to fructose. At the small intestine, an enzyme separates table sugar into its parts, and glucose and fructose are then absorbed. Lactose (milk sugar) is glucose linked to galactose. Only when lactose is broken down by an enzyme at the small intestine are its component parts absorbed. Various vegetables, particularly legumes, contain complex sugars, such as raffinose, that are very resistant to breakdown into the component parts that are absorbable at the small intestine. This accounts for beans' notoriety as a gas producer. The sugar in bread, with the exception of bread made from rice flour, is not always completely absorbed either. This is not due to the sugar but to gluten, a special protein that slows down the time it takes to break complex sugars to simple, absorbable sugars. The complex sugar, waiting in vain for its turn to be broken down, is hurried down the intestinal tract by peristalsis. In the end, it is broken down by colon bacteria. This unbroken complex sugar is not, therefore, utilized as a food, but instead becomes a gas producer.

DEALING WITH FLATULENCE

To treat flatulence, identify all the possible causes, singly or in combination, and eliminate them from the diet. If you are adversely affected by milk or by gluten in bread, be particularly careful to eliminate them from your diet. Try to swallow less air: eat more slowly, do not talk while you eat, do not chew gum, and do not inhale deeply if you smoke. Become aware of swallowing air excessively when you are nervous; substitute deep, calming inhalations through the nose and slow exhalations through the mouth.

An irritable small bowel itself contributes to the malabsorption of sugar. Rest the bowel with a simple, nonirritating diet, and avoid stress. Avoid foods such as legumes, cabbage, whole grains, bran, and pastries, all of which contain complex sugars that are difficult to convert to simple ones. If you are among those for whom milk or other dairy products cause gastric discomfort, you may benefit from taking the enzyme lactase, available in pill form or in pretreated milk, such as Lactaid.

Lactase specifically breaks the lactose sugar down to glucose and galactose, which are then both absorbed. The enzyme alpha-galactosidase, marketed as "Beano," helps break down the linkages of complex sugars in troublesome vegetables such as legumes and cabbage, as well as those sugars in whole grains and bran. Some cookbooks recommend presoaking dried beans overnight, then discarding the soaking water and cooking them in fresh water, claiming that this method eliminates beans' indigestible carbohydrates (ogliosaccharides).

A gas-reducing diet is lactose-free and low in wheat, oats, corn, fiber, and gluten bread. Also avoid artificial sweeteners such as sorbitol and mannitol. Apple and grape juice, raisins, prunes, and bananas are potent gas producers, but orange juice and apricot nectar are virtually gasless. Although fiber is an important part of the diet, it does contain large amounts of unabsorbable carbohydrates; therefore, reduce fiber intake to reduce gas.

Gas-Producing Foods

- Apples/apple juice
- Bananas
- Bran
- Cabbage
- Dairy products
    (for lactase-deficient people)
- Figs
- Grapes/grape juice
- Legumes
- Pastries
- Prunes
- Raisins
- Whole grains

14

Itching: A Delicate Subject

■

A dermatology professor paused during a lecture on itching. "I have never understood," she mused, "why they always torture prisoners with pain. By the time they've made a prisoner want to confess, he passes out. But itching . . . If I were head of an intelligence agency, that is what I would use. Itching drives you crazy. You'll do anything to make it stop."

Particularly annoying is anal itching; that part of the anatomy is quite indelicate to scratch. Sometimes people are so embarrassed by anal itching that they hesitate to consult a physician. They try to stop the itching with an anesthetic ointment, which may, in fact, give some relief. Yet there have also been instances when the ointment caused an allergic reaction that intensified the itching.

Even if an ointment gives relief and causes no additional problems, you might be doing yourself a disservice by masking an important symptom. At its most serious, itching announces the presence of diabetes, leukemia, or other disease. When the disease is treated, the itching goes away.

Anal itching is most commonly caused by rashes due to friction from tight underwear, heat, and excessive sweating—the only condition for which talcum powder is a recommended treatment. Hemorrhoids cause itching when they swell and stretch pain fibers under the skin. Not all hemorrhoids cause itching; very swollen ones cause pain. (Itching is actually mild pain; tickling is mild itching.)

Hemorrhoidal itching can be relieved with cortisone ointment, which should be prescribed by a physician; a "-caine"-derivative anesthetic ointment, provided there is no history of allergy to Novocain or any similar medication; or hot sitz baths. If itching becomes severe, another medical treatment for hemorrhoids may be necessary.

Itching can also be caused by allergic reactions to foods, antibiotics, or other medications; parasites; or skin diseases such as eczema, psoriasis, or friction dermatitis. If there is no discernible cause, doctors often ascribe itching to nervousness or neurosis. Some even treat it in such cases with hypnosis to transfer the itch to a more socially neutral area. Deflecting the itch often obviates it entirely.

PARASITES

Some Egyptologists postulate that living conditions used to be so poor in Egypt because many workers were afflicted with the local parasite and had little energy left for social activism. The schistosomiasis parasite lives in snails in the

Nile River. When the Nile floods, it enriches the soil along its banks with silt and brings the infected snails under soil tillers' bare feet. The upwardly mobile parasite then switches hosts. Modern public health measures in Egypt have reduced this problem considerably.

In every part of the world there are parasites that invade the human body. South America also has a snail parasite; Mexico, an amoeba. In the United States' Deep South, field workers unwittingly pick up hookworm through their bare feet. Pinworm is common among children, who often neglect to wash their hands after bowel movements. If they are thumb suckers, the parasite is recycled. Many a nursery-school teacher has received parasites at the hands of young students.

Most parasites are transmitted through food and water. For example, feasting on rare pork may give you trichinosis. A few parasites, like *Giardia*, may be transmitted through sexual contact.

Some quiet parasites make themselves at home in the intestines without bothering their host too much, but most cause a rash, diarrhea, or itching. Some can cause even more serious trouble if they enter the bloodstream. Most parasites, including pinworms, are so small that they can be seen only in fecal samples through a microscope. Others, such as threadworms, can be seen with the naked eye.

It is not a good idea to reach for an antiworm medication when you have an anal itch. First of all, you may not have worms. More important, if you do have a parasite, it must be identified by a physician and treated with its own specific medication. Parasites rarely go away by themselves. They frequently spread to other members of a family, who should also be examined by a physician. Until you can get to a doctor, applications of witch hazel or calamine lotion to the anus or hot sitz baths can give temporary relief.

ALLERGIES

The fragrant green toilet paper that goes so well with the new shower curtain may also be the reason for the itch you can't seem to get rid of. Or maybe the culprit is the chocolate bar you grab after work every day to cheer you during the crowded bus ride home.

Samuel S. had anal itching "on and off" for 10 years and could not figure out why. His doctor ruled out diabetes, rash, parasites, and skin disease, diagnosing nonspecific pruritus ani (anal itching with no apparent cause). Eventually it dawned on Samuel that he itched only after attending athletic events, the only time he ever ate peanuts. He stopped eating peanuts, and the itch disappeared.

When you find yourself afflicted with anal itching, it may be time to play detective. The "big three" allergens are coffee, any kind of nuts, and chocolate, and you should begin your investigation by regarding these as your main suspects. The "elimination diet" is the best way to track down the villain.

First, avoid eating any of these for two weeks and observe whether the itching subsides. At the beginning of the third week, resume drinking or eating the one you missed most. Perhaps you have been longing for your morning coffee. Drink it in the usual amount, and see if there is a cause-and-effect relationship. Is the itching worse? Or is there no apparent change?

Itching: A Delicate Subject

If coffee does not seem to cause the itching, try one of the remaining suspects, say, chocolate, the next week. Eat it daily. You may continue to drink coffee as well. If chocolate seems to be innocent, try nuts the fifth week.

If none of these appears to be the offending agent, check out other possibilities, such as alcoholic beverages and spicy foods. Itching that is only occasional and especially severe at night can often be linked to what you ate that day. When itching keeps you awake one night, turn on the light and make a list of everything you ate for breakfast, lunch, dinner, and snacks. Omit nothing. Examine the list to notice any foods that are unusual for you. For example, perhaps you dined at a Chinese restaurant instead of the French one you usually choose. An Italian meal may have been very spicy; an Indian curry, fiery. Maybe you sipped red wine instead of your customary Chablis, or ordered Bourbon instead of Scotch.

By avoiding an "unusual" food for two weeks, then eating it daily for one, you might pinpoint the itching's origin.

You may not be allergic to a food at all. Textiles can cause allergic reactions. The "big three" are wool, silk, and synthetics; cotton is the least allergenic fabric. Dye in underwear can also cause itching. Wearing white cotton underwear can eradicate your problem almost instantly.

Nylon panty hose often cause itching. Women should choose only brands with a cotton crotch; better yet, wear cotton underwear underneath.

Allergic reactions may also result from perfumes, scented soaps, dusting powders, lotions, and feminine hygiene deodorant sprays.

Sometimes the prettiest, most expensive brand of toilet paper can be the worst for you. Perfumes, dyes, bleach, and caustic chemicals used to convert rags to toilet paper may be irritating to your skin.

If itching is severe, whatever the cause, do not use toilet paper at all. Substitute cotton balls, first using one moistened with water, then another to pat dry. Make sure the cotton balls are genuine cotton, not rayon or other synthetic balls usually labeled "cosmetic puffs."

Tracking down the cause of an allergy takes time, diligence, and patience. It is important, as you conduct the investigation, not to use anything on the anal area that can aggravate the itch. Analgesic ointments containing a "-caine" derivative can deaden itch temporarily but can sometimes produce an allergic reaction themselves. Witch hazel and calamine lotion can give some relief and are less allergenic. Some people like using a paste of baking soda and water. Petroleum jelly can reduce friction, and hot baths also help.

Next to discovering and eliminating the cause of itching, the best treatment is cortisone. It should be prescribed by a doctor and should not be used for too long. In excess, cortisone can affect the rest of the body as well, producing side effects such as weight gain and puffiness.

Cortisone is usually not effective for itching caused by antibiotics, but this condition usually goes away by itself sometime after antibiotics are discontinued. There can, however, be a delayed reaction to antibiotics, with itching occurring one or two weeks after discontinuing the medication. This itching simply must run its course.

15

Colitis and Diverticulitis

■

While hemorrhoids are one of the most common lower bowel disorders, they are rarely life-threatening or severely restrictive. Other lower bowel problems, however, can cause serious health problems.

COLITIS

Colitis is an inflammation of the large intestine. It may cause bleeding, abdominal cramping, and sporadic, distressingly unpredictable peristaltic contractions. The condition is sometimes temporary and easily cured, or it may be a lifelong affliction with unknown cause and no permanent cure.

Although chronic colitis is an unpleasant condition, people do learn to live with it and have close to normal lives. For example, for one lawyer and avid outdoorswoman, who had developed ulcerative colitis as a teenager, mornings were an especially difficult time. She often needed to spend two hours in the bathroom after breakfast. So she went on camping trips with friends, but instead of sleeping in a tent she stayed at a nearby motel and joined them for hiking and swimming during the day. When job hunting, she chose a position that allowed her to delay arrival at work until midmorning. She also found that reducing emotional anxiety had a beneficial effect on the colitis.

The most common type of colitis, *infectious colitis*, is temporary. Known as *picnic diarrhea*, it is caused by bacteria in contaminated food and can be cured by medication in a couple of weeks (see Chapter 7).

Antibiotic-induced colitis is a toxic reaction to certain antibiotics taken by people who are sensitive to them. Discontinuing the antibiotic usually cures the colitis. Eating yogurt may help prevent antibiotic colitis by preserving the balance of bacteria that normally exist in the colon.

Allergic colitis, caused by allergy to various substances, can be cured by avoiding them. Dairy products are common offenders. But for some people, intolerance of dairy products is not an allergic reaction but an innate bodily deficiency of lactase, an enzyme that promotes the digestion of milk products. Lactase tablets can alleviate this condition, which seems to be most common among black people.

Chemical colitis is caused by directly introducing irritating chemicals—such as strong laxatives, enemas containing turpentine or soap—into the lower intestinal tract. The cure is to discontinue use of the offending chemical (see Chapter 6).

Ischemic colitis, which is relatively rare, is caused by a blood clot blocking a blood vessel that nourishes the intestinal wall. This condition may resolve spontaneously, but sometimes surgery is required, especially if the condition is severe.

Radiation colitis is caused by the implantation of radium needles for treatment of cancer of the cervix in females or cancer of the prostate gland in males, or from external radiation therapy for other conditions.

Colitis can be a side effect of rare systematic illnesses of long duration. Scleroderma, while not a colitis, causes thickening, rigidity, and atrophy of bowel wall tissue. Illnesses such as cancer, anemia, and tuberculosis sometimes cause amyloidosis: waxy substances (amyloids) deposited on the bowel wall. Successful treatment of the primary disease may cure the colitis.

Spastic colitis, or *irritable bowel syndrome,* which has no known cause, is marked by abdominal pain, watery (never bloody) diarrhea and gas, and/or constipation and gas. The condition may occur spontaneously but is more often brought on by emotional stress or occurs after eating. A doctor diagnoses spastic colitis primarily by ruling out other types of colitis, and prescribes fiber supplements or antispasmodic medication to directly restore the intestinal wall's normal muscle contractions. People whose colitis is associated with emotional stress can learn to reduce stress through counseling or meditating. Tranquilizers, taken by prescription and in moderation, can relieve both anxiety and the colitis it causes.

Inflammatory bowel disease (IBD) includes two especially virulent types of colitis: ulcerative colitis and granulomatous colitis. *Ulcerative colitis* is a biphasic disease. Its onset primarily occurs in individuals five to 30 years of age and those age 55 and older. Onset is possible in the intervening years of life but is less common. Some or all of the large intestine's lining is inflamed and patterned by scattered shallow ulcers. The result: bloody diarrhea, abdominal cramping, fever, and weight loss. The medicines cortisone, sulfasalazine, mesalamine, and olsalazine are often effective in treating ulcerative colitis.

But if the condition is long-lasting, complications can include cancer in inflamed tissue, blockage or obstruction of the bowel width from scar tissue, or toxic dilation of the bowel, when part of the bowel suddenly balloons outward, losing its contractile power and blocking feces. These complications may require colectomy, the complete removal of the large intestine. Often the small intestine can be connected to the anus to enable defecation to continue as normally as possible.

Ulcerative colitis affects the bowel's surface membrane. With *granulomatous colitis*, or *Crohn's disease*, the bowel wall's entire thickness is inflamed and thickened with patchy granulelike formations. Crohn's disease can involve any section of the entire gastrointestinal tract from mouth to anus, but most frequently it affects the last part of the small intestine (the ileum) and the colon, usually sparing the rectum.

Crohn's disease causes diarrhea (usually not bloody), weight loss, and abdominal pain. Unexplained anemia or fever is sometimes the first symptom. Fewer ulcers and cancers occur in Crohn's disease than in ulcerative colitis. Crohn's can cause obstruction, abscesses, bowel wall fistulas, and sudden toxic swelling of the bowel. Crohn's can be treated with colectomy. It can also be treated with cortisone or sulfasalazine; which treatment will be effective often depends on the location or severity of the inflammation.

Like ulcerative colitis, Crohn's disease occurs primarily in the teens and early twenties, with a secondary rise in the late fifties. For unknown reasons, both conditions occur more often among Jewish people, males, and Caucasians than among non-Jews, females, and nonwhites. The annual number of ulcerative colitis cases appears stable, but Crohn's disease appears to be on the rise.

DIVERTICULITIS

A diverticulum is a little pouch that balloons out from an inherently weak area in the colon wall, most often in the sigmoid. The condition of having diverticula (more than one diverticulum) is called diverticulosis, and a person may never have any symptoms. Some theorize that the condition called diverticulitis may occur when stool particles get trapped in the pouches and inflammation sets in. The symptoms resemble appendicitis but appear on the left side of the abdomen. Severe inflammation may cause bowel obstruction or perforation and necessitate surgery. Treatment consists of bedrest, antibiotics, antispasmodics, and a diet low in roughage.

16

How a Doctor Treats Fissures, Fistulas, Polyps, and Colon-Rectal Cancer

■

FISSURES

Perhaps the most painful anal malady is the fissure, a crack in the skin and membrane of the anal canal. It is usually caused by exceeding the stretchability limit of the anal sphincter muscles. Pushing too hard and too long with a hard, dry stool or careless insertion of a foreign object can cause tearing on the surface of the skin, at the anal opening, or just inside the anal canal. Acute, deep fissure may occur suddenly, whereas superficial, chronic fissure may cause burning and aching with bowel movements over a period of months.

The fissure, which can be seen by spreading the buttocks, rarely extends farther than a quarter of an inch into the anal canal. If the crack is shallow, hot sitz baths, acetaminophen, and stool softeners will give relief. The fissures will heal within two or three weeks.

But if the fissure has cut through-skin and membrane to deeper tissue or the sphincter muscles, it may require repair through procedures known as internal anal sphincterotomy or anal dilatation. These are ambulatory procedures. Normal activity can usually resume within twenty-four hours.

FISTULAS

A fistula is a tunnel caused by infection. No one knows exactly what causes it, but many doctors suspect that one of the anal glands beneath the dentate line may trap a bit of feces, which irritates surrounding tissue and activates bacteria that eat through the tissue and start an inflammation. When an abscess forms, infection spreads through tissue. The "tunnel infection" may have several tributaries, or branches. A fistula does not always have an external opening. If there is one, it can be as far as an inch or two from the anal opening.

The first sign of a fistula is a throbbing sensation, a foul-smelling discharge that is not bloody, or discovery of its external opening, which may feel like a small protuberance accompanied by swelling and occasional tenderness. Although it is sometimes possible to treat a fistula by draining the infection from within the anal canal, this cannot guarantee that all infection has been caught. In fact, improper or uncontrolled draining can even create another fistula as the infection burrows deeper into the tissue.

A doctor ascertains the extent of a fistula by inserting a flexible silver wire probe into its external opening. In the fourteenth century, John of Arderne invented this diagnostic procedure using a boar's hair as a thread.

The doctor threads the probe through the length of the fistula tunnel, then through the internal opening. At the same time, the doctor places an anoscope inside the canal. When the end of the probe taps the anoscope, the doctor turns the instrument around to see exactly where the fistula's internal opening is and brings the probe tip through.

A fistulectomy, which surgically removes the entire fistulous tract, or tunnel, requires hospitalization. A fistulotomy, which "un-roofs" or opens the fistula to allow drainage of the infection, is an ambulatory procedure. A fistulotomy is appropriate for shorter, superficial fistulas. In a fistulectomy, the fistula tunnel, its external and internal openings, and any tributaries are isolated and removed. The fistulectomy requires hospitalization of about five days. Recovery time is two or three weeks.

POLYPS

A polyp, which is a warty growth, may be a sign of cancer. The smaller a polyp is, the more likely it is to be benign; however, polyps that are at least a quarter of an inch long must always be removed and biopsied. Many benign polyps are considered dormant, with the potential to become cancerous. The longer they stay in the tissue and grow, the greater their chances of becoming malignant.

The presence of polyps should alert the physician to

an acute need for watchfulness. If you have had a polyp, undertake a surveillance program consisting of colonoscopy at regular intervals to detect polyp regrowth or the growth of any new polyps. Discovery through sigmoidoscopy of a polyp low in the intestinal tract may indicate the presence of other polyps higher in the tract, where only colonoscopy would reveal them.

The doctor removes a polyp by snaring it with an electrified wire and drawing tight, cutting the polyp free. This procedure is done in a doctor's office and is painless.

CANCER

Cancer in the anal or rectal canal can appear as a single polyp or a group of polyps. Treatment depends on where and how early the cancer is found.

Low-Lying Cancer

Cancer in the anal canal or lower rectum can sometimes be treated with local excision, chemotherapy, radiation therapy, or laser therapy. With larger cancers, however, the surgeon must remove the anal canal or lower rectum along with the cancer itself. The entire anal area is sewn together, leaving no anal opening. To provide an outlet for feces, the surgeon creates an opening in the abdominal wall called a colostomy, then stitches to it the lowest part of the bowel that remains open and cancer-free. Fecal waste is eliminated into the opening, where it is collected in a disposable colostomy bag. Although the idea of a colostomy can be distressing, most people who have one find they are able to get used to it and to live normal lives. Most hospitals have support groups or counselors to help patients cope with their colostomies.

Higher Cancer

If cancer is found in the middle third of the rectal canal or higher, the anal opening does not need to be closed. The surgeon performs an "anterior resection," removing the cancerous portion of the bowel and sewing together the now open lower part of the colon and the upper end of the rectum. Reconstructing the canal enables the patient to maintain a continuous flow of feces. The colon is sufficiently stretchable to allow the shortened canal to regain normal functioning.

Sometimes, if the area surrounding the cancerous tissue is badly infected, the area must be "rested" to heal infection before the cancer is removed. Feces that pass through and irritate the cancerous part of the bowel are rerouted through a temporary colostomy to go through the abdominal opening into the colostomy bag. This enables the cancer to quiet down and become less inflamed. (More commonly, temporary colostomies are performed when surgery is done to unblock colonic obstruction.) After two or three weeks, the surgeon removes the cancer, disengages the colon from the abdominal wall, and after giving the colon a fresh edge, sews it to the lower part of the rectum. For the first week after surgery, intravenous feeding ensures that feces will not contaminate the stitches holding the two cuts ends of the colon together. After that, bowel function is normal.

17

Sexually Transmitted Diseases

∎

Since the beginning of recorded history, people have often regarded the anus as an erogenous zone. Anal sex was mentioned in the Bible, portrayed on pre-Incan pottery, and extolled in ancient Greece. In the Roman Emire, young lovers often made their coupling an anal affair to preserve the woman's virginity. The night before their wedding, the bridegroom's mother inspected her future daughter-in-law to make sure her hymen was intact. A broken hymen meant a broken engagement.

Today many people—gay men and heterosexual couples—have anal intercourse, for intimacy and pleasure and as a means of birth control. The anus is less stretchable than the vagina, so anal intercourse requires plenty of lubricant and sensitively paced penetration. It is questionable whether anal intercourse can cause or increase one's tendency to develop hemorrhoids. But friction and pressure can irritate existing hemorrhoids and may cause bleeding. Anal intercourse may also make one more susceptible to contracting sexually transmitted diseases (STDs). Human immunodeficiency virus (HIV), the virus that causes acquired immune deficiency syndrome (AIDS), is one STD that is especially thought to have spread quickly through unprotected anal intercourse.

CONDOMS

Using a condom protects against sexually transmitted diseases. Latex condoms provide better protection than animal skin condoms. Do not use petroleum jelly as a lubricant because it can damage the condom and cause it to break. Instead use a lubricant such as K-Y jelly or, even better, a spermicidal jelly that includes nonoxynol-9, a chemical believed to destroy not only sperm but also certain microorganisms, such as HIV, that cause STDs. Some couples use two condoms plus spermicidal jelly for extra protection.

Put on a condom as soon as the penis is erect. Make sure you leave about a half-inch of space at the tip of the condom for semen; before rolling the condom on the rest of the way, squeeze the tip of the condom to press out any air. After intercourse, withdraw right after ejaculating. Hold the condom at the base to prevent it from slipping off and leaking semen into your partner's body. Since even ordinary bacteria in the anus can cause infection in the vagina, care should be taken to change the condom after anal penetration and use a new condom before subsequent vaginal penetration.

TRANSMISSION AND DIAGNOSIS OF STDS

The microorganisms that cause STDs flourish in wet, warm, dark places—the genitals, the anus, the mouth. Hence STDs can be transmitted through unprotected (no condom) anal intercourse, mouth-to-anus sexual contact, or vaginal or oral sexual intercourse.

Unprotected anal intercourse carries a higher likelihood of transmitting STDs because anal fissures, which are small or sizable tears in the anus or within the anal canal, can be caused by overly vigorous or inadequately lubricated penetration. HIV or other microorganisms in an infected person's semen enter the partner's bloodstream through these tears.

Another risky practice is mouth-to-anus contact, through which such diseases as hepatitis B can be spread. Oral-anal sex is safer if a "dental dam" (a rectangle of latex) or a condom (cut to lay flat) is placed on the anus so that the partner's mouth does not actually come into contact with it.

People who have unprotected sex with multiple partners have increased odds of contracting STDs and must be especially conscientious about getting regular physical checkups, including proctological examinations. Do not hesitate to request STD testing; it is crucial to your health, your partner's, and any fetus's. STDs can impair fertility and general health, and be passed on to a fetus. The sooner STDs are diagnosed and treated, the less likely they are to cause permanent damage. Early diagnosis of HIV infection enables a person to receive medication sooner for common viral or bacterial infections that can be serious.

There are no vaccines against STDs, and having once had and treated an STD does not protect you from getting it again if you have unprotected sex with an infected person. STDs are much more common than many people realize. They do not discriminate against rich or poor, male or female, old or young. Nor are STDs something to be ashamed of: they are serious diseases to protect against, and to get diagnosed and treated promptly.

Always inform sexual partners about STDs so they can get diagnosed and treated, too. This is especially important since a person can have an STD but experience no symptoms. With some STDs males have symptoms but females often do not. For example, a man with gonorrhea has a discharge from his penis and feels a burning sensation when he urinates. These symptoms are distressing, but at least they alert him to the need to consult a doctor. His female partner may not be so lucky; while some women with gonorrhea do have symptoms to warn them, others do not.

OVERVIEW OF 13 ANALLY TRANSMITTED STDS

Amebiasis

Amebiasis is caused by a single-celled amoeba that thrives in the gastrointestinal tract. It is spread by oral-anal sex, by bad hygiene, or by ingesting contaminated food and drinking water. Symptoms may not appear for days or even weeks after infection, and include diarrhea (often bloody, with mucus), abdominal pain, and low-grade fever. It is diagnosed through microscopic examination of a stool sample and can be treated with medication.

Chancroid

The chancroid, or "soft chancre," is caused by the microoganism *Haemophilus ducreyi*. It appears as single or multiple soft superficial ulcers on the penis or within the vagina. These ulcers might coalesce (join together). They are accompanied by severe inflammation that results in swelling of inguinal glands in the groin, a condition known as buboes. This can become very painful. Chancroid can be treated with antibiotics. It is especially important to diagnose and treat early; it is believed to be one of the major entry points for HIV spread in Africa.

Chlamydia

One of the most prevalent STDs in the United States today, chlamydia is twice as common as gonorrhea. Chlamydia is often asymptomatic; if any symptoms do occur, usually from one to five weeks after contact, they include burning during urination, vaginal or urethral discharge, pain during intercourse for a woman, and irregular spotting.

Chlamydia is diagnosed through a culture, microscopic examination of a smear of infected tissue, or a blood test for antibodies. Treatment consists of tetracycline or erythromycin antibiotic taken orally. In cases that have gone undiagnosed and untreated for long periods, pelvic surgery may be necessary to remove scar tissue.

Chlamydia can cause sterility and eye infections. It is the most common cause of nongonococcal urethritis in men; infected women can develop infections of the urethra or cervix and pelvic inflammatory disease. Infected newborns may have conjunctivitis, pneumonia, eye infections, or blindness, or be stillborn.

Giardia

The parasite *Giardia* is frequently found in the anus of people who have unprotected anal intercourse. Like other parasites, it causes itching and must be treated with its own specific medication.

Gonorrhea

Gonorrhea causes no symptoms in up to 90 percent of infected women and 10 percent of infected men—statistics that underscore the importance of informing sexual partners if they have been exposed to the disease. When symptoms do occur, they usually appear two to 10 (up to 30) days after infection. Symptoms include white or yellow discharge from the penis, vagina, or anus; pain on urination or defecation, sometimes with drops of pus or blood in urine; a mushroomlike odor from the genital area; pain in the pelvic area or abdomen (especially after menstrual periods); swelling and tenderness near the opening of the vagina. A gonorrheal infection within the anal canal may lodge in an anal gland at the dentate line and form an abscess. Pharyngeal (or throat) gonorrheal infection may cause a sore throat but is usually asymptomatic.

Gonorrhea is diagnosed from a culture from body openings that may have been infected, including the cervix, urethra, rectum, and throat, or microscopic examination of pus from the urethra in males. Chlamydia and gonorrhea often occur simultaneously; both conditions can be treated by combining penicillin and tetracycline.

Untreated gonorrhea may result in pelvic inflammatory disease in women. For both men and women gonorrhea can cause sterility, arthritis, endocarditis, perihepatitis, or meningitis.

Infected newborns may be stillborn or premature and have eye infections or blindness. Routine giving of silver nitrate eye drops after delivery prevents gonorrhea-related eye problems in newborns. Antibiotic eye drops that are less irritating may be substituted, but these are less effective.

Herpes Simplex

The herpes simplex virus, also called herpes type 2 or genital herpes, is a cousin of type 1, which causes cold sores and fever blisters. The virus nestles under the skin around the anus or genitals, forming blisters or bumps. There is a feeling of tenderness, or pain if the sores are open, and one may also have swollen glands, fever, and painful urination. Blisters and other symptoms usually go away by themselves within one to four weeks. But because the virus remains in the body indefinitely, perhaps for life, they can recur, especially during times of stress or illness.

Genital herpes is diagnosed through examination and culture of blisters or sores, or blood tests.

Although there is presently no cure for herpes, a prescription drug, acyclovir, is available as an ointment and as tablets to be taken by mouth. Applying the ointment to the sores can lessen the symptoms' severity. The tablets can also be used to decrease the number of recurrent outbreaks. Hot baths and compresses may relieve symptoms.

During pregnancy, herpes can cause miscarriage or stillbirth. Pregnant women who have active herpes lesions may have to deliver by cesarean section. This helps protect newborns from contracting herpes during childbirth, which can result in severe central nervous system damage or death.

Human Immunodeficiency Virus (HIV)

The HIV virus causes AIDS by bringing about the progressive deterioration of the immune system, rendering one vulnerable to opportunistic infections to which most people uninfected with HIV are resistant. HIV may also attack the central nervous system. The virus remains in the body indefinitely, probably for life.

HIV is spread through unprotected sexual intercourse (anal, vaginal, or oral); through sharing of needles with an HIV-infected drug user; and from a pregnant woman to her fetus. Prior to 1985, HIV was also spread through transfusions of infected blood; since then, blood has been screened for HIV, decreasing but not entirely eliminating the risk.

A person can be infected with HIV and feel healthy, because the virus may not cause any symptoms of AIDS for up to 10 years or even longer after infection. When AIDS does develop, it represents a struggle between HIV and a special white blood cell called the lymphocyte. This cell, made in the bone marrow, travels in the blood to the thymus gland in the neck, where it is modified to become the immune system's major player. This modified cell is now called the *T lymphocyte,* or *helper cell.* When HIV overwhelms these helper cells, AIDS ensues.

AIDS symptoms may include fatigue, fever, weight loss, swollen lymph nodes, persistent diarrhea, thrush, unexplained bleeding, and mental deterioration. Two diseases especially associated with AIDS are Kaposi's sarcoma, a form of cancer that causes dark, purplish, thickened blotches on the skin; and *pneumocystis carinii.*

AIDS attacks the intestinal tract early. The first symptoms may be diarrhea so persistent that people lose as much as 10 percent of their normal body weight. Bacteria and protozoa commonly reside in the lower intestine and cause no problems; AIDS, however, renders one vulnerable to these formerly harmless pathogens, with devastating diarrhea as the result. Diarrhea can also be related to a developing anorectal malignancy from Kaposi's sarcoma, lymphoma, or squamous cell carcinoma; or to infection by such agents as *Cryptosporidia, Mycobacteria, Salmonella, Campylobacter, Chlamydia,* cytomegalovirus, and herpes virus.

Diarrhea due to infection is diagnosed through stool examination and culture, biopsy of the rectal wall lining during sigmoidoscopy, blood tests (immunofluorescence), and viral culture of white blood cells. Diarrhea due to malignancies of the intestinal tract is diagnosed through biopsy of masses seen during sigmoidoscopy and colonoscopy. Early diagnosis is vital. Much diarrhea associated with AIDS can be treated, depending on the cause: herpes with aycyclovir; salmonella, campylobacter, and chlamydia with antibiotics; and temporary remissions for Kaposi's sarcoma through experimental use of interferon and interleukin.

AIDS itself is diagnosed through HIV antibody tests, physical exam, and blood studies to determine the immune system's condition. Although there is no specific cure for AIDS, many opportunistic diseases can be treated.

Lymphogranuloma Venereum

Lymphogranuloma venereum is a sexually transmitted viral infection that can seriously impair elimination. As tissue within the rectum becomes infected, antibodies rush in to heal the infection. Scar tissue that forms may be so thick that the lumen, the space within the rectum, narrows and obstructs the fecal exit route. Antibiotics can sometimes relieve the condition, but often the lumen must be stretched or some fibrous tissue must be cut away with an electric current to allow feces to pass.

Molluscum Contagiosum

A sexually transmitted virus, molluscum contagiosum causes small, pinkish white, waxy-textured polyplike growths in the genital area or on the thighs. It is diagnosed through microscopic examination of a growth and can be treated with freezing (cryotherapy) or by using chemicals or electrical current. If new sores appear, additional treatment is needed.

Shigellosis

Shigellosis is caused by bacteria that thrive in the gastrointestinal tract. It causes severe dysentery; passage of blood, mucus, and pus with feces; abdominal and rectal pain; fever; dehydration; and bowel ulcerations. First symptoms generally appear from 24 to 48 hours after infection. Shigellosis is frequently transmitted through anal to oral sexual contact. It is diagnosed through examination of smears or culture and treated with antibiotics and rehydration. Shigellosis can be serious if it is not treated promptly.

Syphilis

Syphilis is caused by a spirochete, a microorganism. It is a disease of escalating seriousness, with several distinct stages.

From 10 to 90 days after transmission, the first sign of syphilis appears in the form of a chancre. This is a hard, painless pimple or blister that quickly becomes an ulcer. It appears where the spirochete entered the body, usually on the anus or genitals, but sometimes on the lips or mouth. In men, a chancre usually occurs on the upper part of the penis's shaft. People may not be aware of a chancre in the anal opening, cervix, or vagina. The chancre heals by itself within a few weeks, but the disease remains in the system. In some people the chancre never appears, but the disease progresses nevertheless.

If syphilis goes untreated, the second state occurs six to 25 weeks later. One has a feeling of ill health, along with one or more of the following symptoms: a highly infectious rash that characteristically appears on the palms of the hands and the soles of the feet; mucous patches or condyloma warts; spotty hair loss; sore throat; swollen glands; headache; pains in muscles, joints, or long bones; loss of appetite; nausea; constipation; and persistent fever. These conditions can last from four to 12 weeks, then go away by themselves—but the disease is not healed.

Syphilis then enters the latent stage, known in its first four years as the early latent stage and after that as the late latent stage. During this time one is symptom-free. But if untreated, syphilis can advance to its final, devastating stage. Late syphilis can cause tumors in affected organs and damage to the nervous system, heart, brain, and other organs, and may produce insanity, senility, blindness, or paralysis. Syphilis is diagnosed through a blood test to detect antibodies to the spirochete and through microscopic examination of organisms from sores. With latent or late syphilis, it must be diagnosed by testing the cerebral spinal fluid to see if the infection has reached the central nervous system.

Penicillin or certain other antibiotics are effective treatments.

Syphilis passed to fetuses and newborns can damage their skin, bones, eyes, teeth, and liver, and cause stillbirth.

Venereal Warts

Venereal warts—also called genital warts, condyloma acuminata, or HPV—are caused by the human papilloma virus (HPV). Symptoms generally appear from one to three months after transmission. Itching, wartlike growths occur on the anus or genitals (and rarely on the vocal cords). There may be few warts, or so many that they form a velvety mosaic around the anus or genitals. Warts may grow more rapidly if another infection is present or if a woman is pregnant. Venereal warts have a tendency to recur. They are highly contagious; may spread enough to block vaginal, rectal, or throat openings; and may predispose women to cervical cancer.

Diagnosis is through examination, and there is no specific cure. However, warts may be removed by several means, most commonly by application of a prescription chemical, podophyllum, a caustic vegetable compound. Podophyllum is very irritating to normal skin and must be carefully applied to the warts only. About six hours after treatment, take a warm sitz bath for at least 20 minutes to remove any excess medication. Pregnant women should not use podophyllum because it can be absorbed through their skin and may harm the fetus.

Warts can also be removed surgically, by freezing (cryosurgery), or by burning them away with an electrical current. Laser therapy is particularly useful in the management of venereal warts. If warts persist in growing back, a biopsy (testing of warty tissue) may be necessary to rule out cancer. If warts occur on the cervix, a specially trained physician may diagnose them through colposcopy: the use of a colposcope, an instrument that enables a physician to examine the surface of the cervix.

Viral Hepatitis

Viral hepatitis is caused by several viruses: hepatitis A (HAV), hepatitis B (HBV), and hepatitis C (also called non-A non-B). HBV is more commonly transmitted sexually, especially by oral-to-anal sexual contact.

Like many STDs, hepatitis B may be asymptomatic at first. When first symptoms do appear, about three months after transmission, they include flulike symptoms—fever, achiness, and fatigue. Later, hepatitis B can cause dark urine, pale stools, and bodily itching, and progress to jaundice and liver damage. Years after infection, some HBV carriers develop liver cancer, which is often fatal.

HBV is diagnosed through examination and blood test. HBV vaccine prevents an individual from contracting the disease. Injection of immune serum globulin shortly prior to or after exposure may prevent or reduce the severity of symptoms. Rest, a restricted diet, and avoidance of alcohol are important in recuperating from infection.

18

Toilet Training: Helping Children Develop Healthy Bowel Habits

■

Learning to use a potty instead of a diaper is a milestone in children's lives. The new skill proves that they are growing up, not babies anymore. Both children and parents feel proud of this accomplishment. It affirms children's increasing maturity and their proficiency at mastering the necessary physical and social skills of adulthood.

Toilet training provides parents with an opportunity to help children develop healthy bowel habits and attitudes that will help protect them against hemorrhoids, constipation, and other bowel problems for a lifetime. Parents should do some soul searching about their own feelings about the elimination process, and try to avoid transferring any anxiety or tension about daily bowel movements to their impressionable children.

The proper age for toilet training varies widely among

children. Many parents begin encouraging children to "sit on the toilet like a big girl" at about a year and a half, but the right time to begin depends on the child's own physical and emotional readiness. Do not get drawn into a competitive spirit about which child gets toilet-trained first: your own or your neighbor's. Keep things in perspective by remembering one grandmother's reassuring wit: "Don't worry, your child will certainly be toilet trained by the time she goes to college!"

The defecation reflex in infants is simple and direct. When food enters the stomach, the colon contracts, and feces enter the rectum and anal canal. At first infants have no control over when stool is passed and are unaffected by extraneous factors such as time or place. As children grow older, they learn that defecation can be suppressed at will to suit caprice or the demands of schedule or household. Then toilet training can begin.

A RELAXED APPROACH

The key to successful toilet training is to keep the process tension-free and to let children set the pace. Relaxed parents help children regard toilet training as an opportunity to identify with their parents and to develop good feelings about authority and organization. Parents should praise children for using the potty or toilet, but not offer material rewards such as candy or gifts. Remember that you want children to respond to *internal* impulses, not external incentives. By the same token, be easygoing, not punitive, when children "mess." It takes children time to become accident-free; even toilet-trained children occasionally lapse when they are too busy, excited, or distracted to remember to use the bathroom. Reassure the child by saying, "That's okay. These things happen sometimes."

Have a potty available, but if a child balks at using it, don't insist. Calmly and confidently say, "That's okay. You'll use it when you are ready." Since the point of toilet training is to increase children's control of their bowels, let children take the lead in readiness. After all, throughout their lives it is not parents who tell them when to use the bathroom, but rather body signals. Encourage children to become aware of "the call of nature"—the feeling that their bodies are "telling" them that it is time to urinate or defecate.

Make sure you discuss your approach to toilet training with children's regular babysitters or caregivers so that children get consistent messages. One mother was appalled upon arriving at her son's day-care center to see the teacher offer her son a piece of chocolate while he sat on the potty. The teacher said that other parents had instructed her to "bribe" their children. The mother explained that eating should be a very separate activity from defecating, and that she wanted her child to use the toilet because his body told him to do so—not because he would get a sweet from the teacher. The teacher readily acquiesced to the mother's wishes.

TOILET TRAINING: AN EMOTIONAL EXPERIENCE

If parents do not hurry toilet training, children will respond naturally to this tension-free approach, growing up sensitive to their own body.

Parents who are tense and anxious about toilet training may make the act of defecation so fraught with emotional overtones that a child develops unhealthy bowel habits. If children are coaxed to "produce" for Daddy, Mommy, Aunt Martha, and so on, they might become so eager to please that they push very hard to have a bowel movement even if feces are not forthcoming. They may suffer from hemorrhoids in later life from pushing so hard.

Sometimes, too, intense parental pressure transforms toilet training into a power struggle. Young children assert their will by stubbornly withholding feces, refusing to defecate upon parental command. Such children may suffer chronic constipation and hemorrhoids later in life. Parents who are overly concerned about the regularity of children's bowel movements may be conveying the message that children are not really innately capable of defecating successfully on their own. It is a way of saying that children "aren't good enough." The fussed-over child may be prodded and coaxed and introduced to enemas and laxatives at a young age. When such children grow up, they continue to obsess over regularity and to use these aids.

HELPING CHILDREN DEVELOP HEALTHY BOWEL HABITS

Healthy bowels are created by a worry-free environment, allowing time to respond to the gastrocolic reflex, and proper diet.

Plan Ahead

Since breakfast and dinner trigger the gastrocolic reflex, guide children to use the toilet after these meals. Children who learn at a young age to allow time for sitting on the toilet after breakfast and dinner are more likely to be regular, unconstipated, and free of hemorrhoids as adults.

Of course, this works only if you don't have to rush children out of the house. Time pressure will force them to suppress the "call of nature" in order to get to day care or school on time. Awaken children early enough so they have time for a bowel movement after breakfast.

Eat Well/Eliminate Well

Give children plenty of raw vegetables, whole-grain bread, and bran or wheat-germ cereals. The sugar-coated processed cereals marketed to children do not usually produce adequate roughage and may also produce dental caries.

At snack time, teach children to reach for a piece of fruit instead of cookies, potato chips, or other highly processed, nonnutritive foods. If you refuse to buy these foods, children will be less likely to develop the junk food habit. On a low shelf in the refrigerator, keep easy-to-open containers of carrot sticks, slices of cucumber and green or red pepper, chunks of crispy lettuce, raw green beans, and steamed then chilled vegetables. Cut cored apples into rings and slice oranges into smile-shape wedges. Children enjoy helping to make fruit salads. Even young children can stir with a wooden spoon, toss in a handful of grapes (cut in half for children under three), and fetch bananas from the kitchen counter. In the cupboard, let children help themselves to whole-grain crackers, croutons, raisins, and dried prunes.

Children should learn to drink plenty of fluids, especially water, which flushes out the kidneys and bladder and helps prevent constipation. They can also drink wholesome fruit or vegetable juices, but not soft drinks or "juice drinks" that contain only a small percentage of juice. Teach children to be careful shoppers by pointing out (with suitable disdain!) why you won't buy those products. Milk is important in children's diets but should not be drunk to excess. It is a low-residue food and contains calcium, which in very high amounts can be constipating.

The Myth of "Regularity"

Contrary to popular belief, a daily bowel movement is not essential. Many normal children get along with a stool every second or third day. *Normal* means what is normal for a particular individual; people's defecation patterns are as unique as their personalities. Do *not* give children laxatives, suppositories, or enemas unless prescribed by a physician. These products only teach children dependence and highlight the bowel movement as something to worry about. If given to an infant, these products can impede development of normal functioning.

Another myth is that a constipated rectum gives off a "toxin." Discomfort from constipation is caused by the mechanical distension of the rectum from feces, not from absorption of any toxic substance. Defecation relieves discomfort.

If a child does become temporarily constipated, the best treatment is none at all. A bowel movement will usually come on by itself in a day or two. Sometimes constipation coincides with other illnesses, in which case treat the illness but do not resort to laxatives or enemas for the constipation.

Consult a physician if constipation is chronic. This is usually due to a faulty diet or poor bowel habits.

Infrequent or difficult evacuation of feces can place a terrible strain on children four months to three years of age. Generally, bottle-fed babies tend to have more of a problem with less frequent, firmer stools than a baby who is breastfed. This may be due to the higher calcium content in cow's milk. Boiling milk can also have a constipating effect.

Infants can, on occasion, go for 48 hours or even longer without a stool and experience no discomfort. If a healthy baby has gone longer than this, however, many pediatricians recommend giving the baby half a teaspoon of milk of magnesia for relief. Adding a little brown sugar to a baby's formula is another way to overcome stool infrequency. When an infant begins to take solid foods that have more residue, the infrequency of stool corrects itself—unless parents have habitually given the baby suppositories, laxatives, or enemas.

19

Anorectal Disorders in Children

∎

Most anorectal disorders in children occur between the ages of four months and two years. The reason for this is structural. Until a child's third year, the anus and rectum lie in a straight line without any bends. They are insecurely attached to the lower end of the spine (the sacrum and coccyx), which acts as a bracing column and which is also straight at that age. After the third year, the sacrum and coccyx bend forward, forming a bony hollow in which the anal canal and lower rectum lie, now curved to fit into the new shape of the spine. They also form more snug attachments to the spine to strengthen their position in the bony hollow.

If a baby puts a great deal of strain on the anorectal canal from constipation or diarrhea, the straight, immature canal, improperly braced and supported, is unduly stretched. Common disorders that result, in order of frequency, include anal fissure, abscess and fistula, and prolapse or procidentia. Hemorrhoids are rare because it takes a long period of straining to cause them.

ANAL FISSURE

A baby or child who stops moving his or her bowels or screams in pain during a bowel movement may have an anal fissure, a crack in the skin around the anal opening. In the very young, fissures are usually superficial and heal with the help of an anesthetic ointment. Dilate the anal opening with your finger when applying the ointment to the fissure.

In a child three years or older, the fissures may be deep, and fissurectomy may be recommended. If the fissure was caused by constipation or diarrhea, that condition must be treated as well.

Fissures may also be caused by a child inserting an object into the anus. Children have been known to insert a wide variety of items into body openings, including mouth, ears, nose, vagina, and anus. Doctors have removed from the anal canal such items as thermometers, jacks, nuts, raisins, and other small objects. These objects may rise high into the rectum, as high as the sigmoid colon or beyond. Small objects may come out with the stool. Sharp objects such as pins can lodge in the wall of the anal canal and cause tremendous pain. An abscess may form.

A doctor removes objects from the rectum or anal canal by using the snare device on a sigmoidoscope—a prong that can hook onto an item and draw it out. Surgery is usually not necessary.

ANAL ABSCESS

In the infant an anal abscess usually starts in the anal glands at the anal canal's dentate line. The abscess often extends and burrows outward to form a fistula, a tunnellike infection. Symptoms are a steady, throbbing pain, irritability, sleeplessness, and discomfort in the sitting position. The only cure for a fistula is surgical removal of infected tissues.

PROLAPSE OR PROCIDENTIA

A protrusion from a child's anal opening is usually a prolapse, if the membrane lining the rectum is loosened, or procidentia, if the entire thickness of the anorectal wall has sagged. These conditions are caused solely by too much strain being placed on the poorly supported anus and rectum, forcing the lining or wall thickness downward to emerge through the anal opening.

Prolapse is treated with an injection of phenol in oil or quinine in urea, which "glues" the lining back to the rectal wall. Procidentia can also be treated this way but on occasion must be corrected surgically. A silver wire is inserted under the skin to act as a "drawstring" around the anal opening. The wire is kept in place for about six weeks, then removed.

Children with anal disorders should be referred to a proctologist or a pediatric gastroenterologist, who examines children exactly the same way as adults, only with smaller instruments.

BIRTH DEFECTS

Proctologists also handle far less common problems in infants. For example, in one out of every 3,000 to 4,000 infants an anorectal birth defect occurs, for no known reason. The anal canal may not have an opening but be covered by a membrane that must be perforated. In a more severe defect, the rectal pouch ends blindly some distance above the anal opening and may even communicate with the vagina or urinary tract, not with the anal canal at all. A congenital nerve disorder called Hirschsprung's disease may prevent an infant from moving his or her bowels. All these conditions can be corrected surgically.

TUMORS AND POLYPS

Infants and children also sometimes develop tumors and other growths, primarily polyps. The most common symptom of a growth is painless bleeding from the anal opening, either daily or at intervals of weeks or even months. If a growth is large, it may interfere with normal functioning and cause abdominal discomfort and diarrhea.

Sometimes a parent may notice a mass protruding from a child's anus. This may be a polyp that has broken off by itself. Such "self-amputations" occur frequently in children but rarely in adults.

Discovery of one polyp may suggest the presence of others. If many are found, the condition is known as polyposis. If this occurs in a young person in the second decade of life, it is likely to be found in other members of the family, too, and is known as familial polyposis. Such a family may develop cancer at an unusually early age.

INFLAMMATORY BOWEL DISEASE (IBD)

In children and adolescents IBD is being recognized with increasing frequency. Pediatric IBD usually starts between 10 and 19 years of age. Two types of IBD, ulcerative colitis and granulomatous colitis (Crohn's disease), present special problems in children that are not seen in adults (see Chapter 15).

In ulcerative colitis, the peak incidence occurs in teenagers and young adults. Rectal bleeding is not as common in young people as in adults. Diarrhea, though, is common in both age groups. Ulcerative colitis may start in children in three different ways. Over half of children will have slow, insidious starts: vague abdominal pain, nausea and vomiting, fever, weight loss, joint pains, and occasional nonbloody diarrhea accompanied by growth failure. A smaller group of children will have a dramatic onset with the sudden appearance of bloody diarrhea, fever, and abdominal cramping. The last group will have the severest onset with all the symptoms of the second group but with the appearance of a condition known as *toxic megacolon*, which occurs when a segment of the colon suddenly balloons out, loses its peristaltic activity, and halts the passage of feces. Stool stagnates and inflammation, fever, and delirium occur. Immediate surgery is required.

Crohn's disease primarily occurs in adults between the ages of 20 to 35 and 55 to 75. However, it is important to know about its incidence in children, since its symptoms are often hidden. In Crohn's disease, abdominal pain and diarrhea are more common than rectal bleeding. Children may bleed with diarrhea twice as commonly as adults with this disease.

Children have many symptoms that are not related to the colon. For instance, fever, anal fistulas, abscess, anemia, and joint pains may precede by years the onset of intestinal complaints. Therefore the combination of fever, abdominal pain, weight loss, anal abscesses, fistulas, growth failure, or joint pains should alert the parent and doctor to the presence of IBD in children.

Nutrition is a key factor in the treatment of IBD. Adequate calories, protein, carbohydrates, fat, and trace minerals (such as zinc) are essential for growth. Increased calories and nutrients can be supplied by special formulas. The medicine Azulfidine (sulfasalazine) helps relieve symptoms when given with folic acid. Corticosteroids are used to treat acute symptoms when Azulfidine has not been beneficial, or when symptoms are severe. Other medications used to relieve symptoms include metronidazole, 6-mercaptopurine, and antibiotics.

When IBD becomes intractable and life-threatening, surgery is needed. Toxic megacolon, massive hemorrhage, and the risk of malignancy are some indications for surgery. Surgery for ulcerative colitis is usually curative. Surgery for Crohn's disease is only palliative because of the high likelihood that the disease will recur.

INTUSSUSCEPTION

Intussusception is an obstruction of the intestine resulting from one section of the bowel telescoping into its adjacent segment. The condition can be compared to a collapsible drinking cup, or to a trouser leg that hangs over its cuff. When such obstruction occurs, bowel contents cannot pass through either partially or completely, and constipation occurs. Telescoping may be caused by the tugging of a large polyp attached to the bowel wall, by an inherited weakness of a segment of the wall, or by the absence of nerves in a segment of the wall.

Intussusception usually occurs at the ileocecal valve, at the beginning of the large intestine. It occurs mostly in young children and at first may be difficult to diagnose. Before obstruction of the bowel is complete, symptoms may include persistent vomiting, which may eventually become fecal; abdominal cramplike pain; abdominal swelling that during examination may feel like a sausagelike bulkiness; and jellylike bleeding from the rectum. Intestinal obstruction can be fatal if it is not relieved promptly.

Fortunately, intussusception can be treated nonsurgically, especially if it is diagnosed early. A doctor can often disengage the telescoped bowel by using a barium enema and gently massaging the abdomen. The controlled force of the enema can straighten out the bowel wall. A doctor can also decompress the bowel by using a nasal suction apparatus, a tube inserted through the nose, down past the stomach into the small intestine. A suction machine attached to the tube reduces vomiting and gas. If neither enema nor suction works, the condition must be corrected surgically.

Index

Abscesses, 22, 25, 27, 124, 125
Acetaminophen, 21, 27, 60
Acyclovir, 107, 109
Aerosol sprays, 59
AIDS (acquired immune deficiency syndrome), 102, 108–109
Alcoholic beverages, 73, 87
Allergic colitis, 90
Allergies, 24, 27, 84, 86–88
Amebiasis, 104
American Cancer Society, 3
Amyloidosis, 91
Anal canal, 11
Anal dilatation, 96
Anal intercourse, 101–103
Anal opening, 9–11
Anal sphincter muscles, 9, 10, 20, 53, 75
Anatomy, 9–13
Anesthetic agents, 58, 60, 83, 84, 88
Animal protein, 3, 73, 74
Anorectal disorders in children, 123–29

Anoscopes, 32, 63, 97
Anterior resection, 99
Antibiotic-induced colitis, 90
Antibiotics, 88
Antidiarrheal medications, 46–47
Antimicrobial medications, 46
Appendix, 12, 13, 41
Ascending colon, 13
Astringents, 58
Atropine, 46, 47, 60
Attapulgite, 46
Azulfidine, 128

Banding method of treatment, 65
Barium enema X ray, 34–35
Baths, 7, 21, 24, 27, 56, 60, 68, 84
Beans, 79, 81
Becker, Ernest, 16–17
Belladonna, 47, 58, 60
Benzocaine, 58
Birth defects, 126
Bismuth, 46, 58
Bleeding, 7, 21–22, 26–27, 60
Boric acid, 59

Bowel. *See* Colon
Bowel habits, changes in, 22–23, 26–27
Bowel movements
  forcing, 15, 16, 55, 118
  postponing, 2, 12, 55, 60, 69–72
  toilet training, 12, 115–21
Bran, 2, 54, 72–75, 119
Breathing
  during physical exertion, 15–16
  while on toilet, 17
Buboes, 105
Buttock press, 27, 75–76

"-caine" derivatives, 58, 60, 84
Calamine lotion, 25, 27, 86, 88
Campylobacter, 109
Cancer. *See* Colon cancer; Rectal cancer
Carbon dioxide, 78
Castor oil, 41
Cecum, 13
Celsus, 63–64
Cereals, bran, 72–74, 119
Chancroid, 105
Chemical additives, 3, 73, 74
Chemical colitis, 90
Children
  anorectal disorders in, 123–29
  constipation and, 120–21
  toilet training, 12, 115–21
Chlamydia, 105, 109
Chocolate, 86
Coal-tar products, 41
Coccyx, 123
Codeine, 47
Coffee, 73, 74, 86
Colace, 40
Colectomy, 92
Colitis, 41, 88–93
Colon, 9, 71
  anatomy of, 12–13
Colon cancer
  early detection of, 30
  prevalence of, 2–3
  symptoms of, 21, 22, 27, 28
  treatment for, 99
Colonoscopes, 32, 34, 35
Colonoscopy, 31, 34, 98
Colostomy, 98–99
Colposcopy, 113
Complex sugars, 79–80
Condoms, 102
Condyloma acuminata, 112–13
Constipation, 2, 22–23
  causes of, 37–38
  children and, 120–21
  elderly and, 51–53
  emotional causes for, 17
  enemas, 38–39, 52, 118, 120, 121
  intussusception, 38, 54, 129
  laxatives, 2, 40–42, 50–52, 54, 118, 120, 121
  pregnancy and, 49
  stool softeners, 21, 40, 52, 57, 60
Corticosteroids, 128
Cortisone, 61, 84, 88, 92–93
Crohn's disease, 91, 92–93, 127–128
Cryosurgery, 65–66, 112

Defecation
  attitudes toward, 16–17
  changes in habits, 22–23, 26–27
  forcing, 15, 16, 55, 118
  postponing, 2, 12, 55, 60, 69–72
  regularity, 2, 37, 72, 118, 120
Denial of Death, The (Becker), 16–17
Dentate line, 9, 11, 12
Descending colon, 12, 13
Diabetes, 24, 27
Dialose, 40
Diarrhea, 22–23
  causes of, 43–44
  preventing and treating, 45–47
  as symptom of AIDS, 108–109
  traveler's, 44–45

Index

Diet, 2, 3, 23, 38
  for children, 119–20
  diarrhea and, 47
  elderly and, 54
  elimination, 86–87
  gas-reducing, 80–81
  improving, 72–75
  during pregnancy, 50
Digestive system, 9
Diphenoxylate, 46
Discharge, 22, 26–27
Diverticulitis, 41, 93
Doxycycline, 46

Eczema, 84
Elderly, 51–54
Electric current method of treatment, 65, 67, 112–13
Elevations, 25
Elimination diet, 86–87
Embarrassment, 1
Emotional stress, 23, 24, 27, 37, 91
Endoscopes, 32, 34
Enemas, 38–39, 52, 118, 120, 121
Ephedrine, 58, 60
Exercise, 55
  breathing during, 15–16
  elderly and, 54
  importance of, 75–76

Fabrics, allergenic, 87
Fat, 3
Fecal impaction, 53
Fetal current, 13
Fissurectomy, 124
Fissures, 20–21, 27, 95–96, 103, 124
Fistulas, 21, 22, 25, 27, 63, 64, 96–97, 125
Fistulectomy, 97
Flatulence, 73, 77–81
Folic acid, 128
Food-associated diarrhea, 44, 45
Freezing method of treatment, 65–66
Friction dermatitis, 84

Fructose, 79
Fruits, 2, 54, 72–74, 119

Galactose, 79, 80
Gallstones, 23
Gas, 73, 77–81
Gastrocolic reflex, 38, 71–72, 117–19
Gastroscopes, 32
Genital warts, 112–13
Giardia, 85, 106
Glaucoma, 47, 60
Glucose, 79, 80
Gluten, 79, 81
Gonorrhea, 104, 106–107
Granulomatous colitis, 91, 92–93, 127–28

Hemorrhoidal plexus, 5
Hemorrhoids
  anal intercourse and, 101
  causes of, 15–17
  constipation and. *See* Constipation
  defined, 5–7
  diarrhea and. *See* Diarrhea
  elderly and, 51–54
  heredity and, 15
  in history, 63–64
  pregnancy and, 49–50
  prevention of, 55, 69–76
  self-care of. *See* Self-care
  symptoms of. *See* Symptoms
  treatment of, 64–68
Henry V, King of England, 64
Hepatic flexure, 13
Hepatitis, 23, 45
Hepatitis B, 103, 113
Herbal laxatives, 41
Heredity, hemorrhoids and, 15
Herpes simplex, 107, 109
Hippocrates, 63–65
Hookworm, 85
Human immunodeficiency virus (HIV), 102, 103, 105, 108–109

Human papilloma virus (HPV), 112–13
Hydrogen, 78

Ileum, 92
Immunofluorescence, 109
Imodium, 46, 47
Incontinence, 53
Infection, 96–97
Infectious colitis, 90
Inflammation, 21, 96
Inflammatory bowel disease (IBD), 22, 27, 91–92, 127–28
Injection method of treatment, 64–65
Interferon, 109
Interleukin, 109
Internal anal sphincterotomy, 96
Intrauterine devices (IUDs), 30
Intussusception, 38, 54, 129
Irritable bowel syndrome, 91
Ischemic colitis, 90–91
Itching, 24–27, 61, 83–88

John of Arderne, 64, 97

Kaolin, 46
Kaopectate, 46
Kaposi's sarcoma, 108, 109
Kegel exercises, 76
Knee-chest position, 56
K-Y jelly, 57, 102

Lactase, 80, 90
Lactobacillus culture, 47
Lactose, 79, 80
Large intestine. *See* Colon
Laser method of treatment, 65, 66–68, 113
Laxatives, 2, 40–42, 50, 118
  children and, 120, 121
  elderly and, 51–52, 54
Lidocaine, 58
Lomotil, 46
Loperamide, 46, 47
Louis XIV, King of France, 64

Lumen, 12, 109–10
Lymphogranuloma venereum, 109–10

Meat, 2, 73, 74
Menthol, 59
Mercury compound, 59
Mesalamine, 92
Methane, 78
Milk, 120
Milk of magnesia, 41, 121
Mineral oil, 41
Molluscum contagiosum, 110

Nitrogen, 78
Nonoxynol-9, 102
Normal stool, 23
  changes from, 23–24, 26–27
Novocaine, 60, 84
Nursing homes, 52, 53
Nutrition. *See* Diet
Nuts, 86

Olsalazine, 92
Oral-anal sex, 103, 104
Osmotic pressure, 39
Over-the-counter preparations, 19–20, 57–61
Oxygen, 78

Pain, 7, 20–21, 26–27
Panty hose, 87
Papillae, 11
Parasites, 22, 24, 27, 45, 59, 84–86
Paregoric, 46, 47
Paulus Aegineta, 64
Pectin, 46
Pelvic inflammatory disease, 105, 106
Pepto-Bismol, 46
Peristaltic contractions, 23
Petroleum jelly, 25, 27, 57, 58, 60, 88, 102
Pharyngeal gonorrheal infection, 106
Phenylephrine, 58

Index

Physiologic salt solution, 39
Picnic colitis, 90
Pinworm, 85
Pneumocystis carinii, 108
Podophyllum, 112
Polyposis, 126–27
Polyps, 25, 97–98, 126–27
Pregnancy, 16, 49–50
Prevention of hemorrhoids, 55, 69–76
Procidentia, 25, 53, 125
Proctology, 64
Prolapse, 25, 53, 125
Protrusions, 25–27
Prunes, 50
Psoriasis, 84
Psychotherapy, 17

Radiation colitis, 91
Raffinose, 79
Raw fruits and vegetables, 2, 54, 72–74, 119
Reagan, Ronald, 34
Rectal cancer
  early detection of, 30
  prevalence of, 2–3
  symptoms of, 21, 22, 27, 28
  treatment for, 98–99
Rectal examination, 29–35
Rectum, 9, 12, 123
  common symptoms of problems, 20–28
Referred pain, 20
Refined foods, 2, 3, 72
Regularity, 2, 37, 72, 118, 120
Resorcinol, 59
Roughage, 2, 3, 55, 60, 72, 119

Sacrum, 123
Salmon, Frederick, 64
Salmonella, 45, 109
Scleroderma, 91
Scopolamine, 47
Self-care, 1, 2, 52, 55–61
  knee-chest position, 56
  over-the-counter preparations, 19–20, 57–61

sitz baths, 7, 21, 24, 56, 60, 68, 84
stool softeners, 21, 40, 52, 57, 60
wiping, 57
Sexually transmitted diseases (STDs), 22, 27, 101–13
  amebiasis, 104
  chancroid, 105
  chlamydia, 105
  condoms and, 102
  giardia, 106
  gonorrhea, 104, 106–107
  herpes simplex, 107
  human immunodeficiency virus (HIV), 102, 103, 108–109
  lymphogranuloma venereum, 109–110
  molluscum contagiosum, 110
  shigellosis, 110
  syphilis, 110–12
  transmission and diagnosis of, 103–104
  venereal warts, 112–13
  viral hepatitis, 113
Shigellosis, 110
Sigmoid colon, 12
Sigmoidoscopes, 32–34
Sigmoidoscopy, 31–33, 98
Simple sugars, 79
Sitz baths, 7, 21, 24, 27, 56, 60, 68, 84
Skin disease, 24, 27
Small intestine, 13, 79, 92
Soft drinks, 73, 74, 120
Soilage, 25–27, 53
Spastic colitis, 91
Spermicide, 102
Spicy foods, 87
Splenic flexure, 12
Stenosis, 67
Stools, change from normal, 23–24, 26–27
Stool softeners, 21, 27, 40, 52, 57, 60
Stress, 23, 24, 27, 37, 91
Sucrose, 79

Sugar, 74
Sugar ingestion, 79–81
Sulfasalazine, 92, 93, 128
Suppositories, 52, 58, 59, 120, 121
Surgery, 65, 67–68
Swelling, 24, 26–27
Symptoms, 7, 19–28
    bleeding, 21–22, 26–27
    change from normal stool, 23–24, 26–27
    change in bowel habits, 22–23, 26–27
    discharge, 22, 26–27
    elevations, 25–27
    itching, 24–27, 83–88
    pain, 20–21, 26–27
    protrusions, 25–27
    soilage, 25–27
    swelling, 24, 26–27
Syphilis, 21, 25, 110–12

Tampons, 30
Tannic acid, 58
Tension, 23
Threadworms, 85
Thrombosis, 7
TMP-SMX, 46
Toilet paper, 86, 87–88
Toilet training, 12, 115–21
Toxic megacolon, 127, 128
Tranquilizers, 91
Transverse colon, 12–13
Traveler's diarrhea, 44–45
Treatment of hemorrhoids, 64–68
Trichinosis, 85
Tumors, 22, 23, 126
Tunnel infection, 96–97, 125

Ulceration, 21
Ulcerative colitis, 91–93, 127–28
Underwear, 84, 87
Unprocessed bran, 72–73

Valsalva maneuver, 15
Valves of Houston, 9, 12, 33, 71
Vegetables, 2, 54, 72–74, 119
Venereal warts, 112–13
Viral hepatitis, 113
Vitamins A and D, 59
Volvulus, 38, 54

Water, 55, 73, 74, 75, 120, 121
Wheat germ, 74
White flour, 74
Whole-grain bread, 74, 119
Wiping, 57
Witch hazel, 25, 27, 86, 88
Worms, 85

Yeast-cell extracts, 59
Yoga, 16
Yogurt, 47, 90

Zinc compounds, 58